ASM
POCKET GUIDE TO
Clinical Microbiology

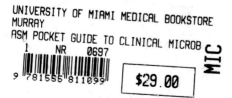

ASM

POCKET GUIDE TO

Clinical Microbiology

Patrick R. Murray, Ph.D., ABMM

Professor, Pathology and Medicine
Co-Director, Clinical Microbiology Laboratories
Washington University Medical Center
St. Louis, Missouri

ASM Press
Washington, D.C.

Copyright © 1996 American Society for Microbiology
1325 Massachusetts Avenue, N.W.
Washington, DC 20005

Library of Congress Cataloging-in-Publication Data

Murray, Patrick R.
  ASM pocket guide to clinical microbiology / Patrick R.
Murray.
    p.   cm.
  ISBN 1-55581-109-4 (softcover)
  1. Medical microbiology—Handbooks, manuals, etc.
I. Title.
  [DNLM: 1. Microbiology—handbooks.
2. Microbiological Techniques—handbooks.
3. Antibiosis—handbooks.   4. Microbial Sensitivity
Tests—handbooks.   QW 39 M983a 1996]
QR46.M92   1996
616′.01—dc20
DNLM/DLC
for Library of Congress   96-4638
                                                              CIP

10 9 8 7 6 5 4 3 2

*To Julie, Tim, David, and Melissa
whose questions and support have been
my impetus to reduce complex concepts
to practical guidelines*

Contents

SECTION 4
Specimen Processing   81

SECTION 5
Microbial Identification   115

SECTION 6
Antimicrobial Agents and Susceptibility Testing   185

SECTION 7
Immunodiagnostic Tests   *221*

SECTION 8
Notifiable Infectious Diseases   *251*

Preface

In the formative years of our education as clinical microbiologists, many of us reduce our learning process to one simple question: "What do we really need to know?" As we mature and expand our knowledge, we rationalize our search for "really important information" by segregating knowledge into what we can recite at the slightest provocation and what we leave to be found in reference books. Most of us feel comfortable with this approach. Unfortunately, many answers to important questions have been misfiled in my brain and are now retrievable only from the reference books in my office or library. While this does not pose a problem when I am in my office, it is a problem when I am in the clinical laboratory or a conference or when I am approached by a medical colleague in a hospital corridor. My failings are not unique but are shared by many of my medical counterparts. How many times have you seen physicians walk down a corridor with their pockets full of guidebooks detailing all the important information in pharmacology, infectious diseases, or internal medicine? It was from this simple observation and the realization that my memory is never as good as it needs to be, that this *Pocket Guide to Clinical Microbiology* was conceived.

From the first discussions of this *Pocket Guide,* a few simple principles shaped its development. First, from a practical perspective, it had to fit into the pocket of a laboratory coat; hence the small size. A pocket guide is never valuable unless it is used. If it sat on my office shelf, then it would compete with the American Society for Microbiology (ASM) *Clinical Microbiology Procedures Handbook,* the ASM *Manual of Clinical Microbiology,* my four-volume edition of *The Prokaryotes,* my two-volume *Mandell's Principles and Practice of Infectious Diseases,* Lorian's *Antibiotics in Laboratory Medicine,* and the dozen or so other reference books I open frequently. Second, information in a pocket guide must be organized to be easily retrievable. If I can walk to my office faster than it takes to find the answer in the guidebook, then the book is not useful. For this reason, this pocket guide is subdivided into eight sections, and the information is presented in tables and charts with minimal reliance on textual comments. Finally, the information that I really need to know must be in the guide. Obviously, each microbiologist will have a different idea of what needs to be in this book. I have selected information on the basis of my experience as the director of a major medical laboratory, a teacher of laboratory medicine residents and fellows in microbiology and infectious diseases, and the author of many scientific research articles and reference books.

In my first undertaking of this nature, I can be certain that some topics will hit the target and others will sail wide. However, I feel that the future success and growth of this *Pocket Guide to Clinical Microbiology* will be determined by each person who uses it. My commitment and ASM's are to develop a resource for clinical microbiologists that will extend the tradition of excellence founded in the *Manual of Clinical Microbiology* and maintained in the other clinical microbiology texts published by ASM. To that end I ask that you, the reader and user of this book, tell me what is good, what is bad, what should be eliminated, and what should be added. It is only by incorporating this input, that future editions of this book will fulfill the promise in which this first edition was conceived.

As in any undertaking, many individuals deserve to be recognized. First, I thank John Washington, who was my preceptor when I was a fellow at the Mayo Clinic. John was critically important in shaping my foundation as a clinical microbiologist. I also thank the supervisors, medical technologists, and technicians who have worked in my laboratory, particularly Joan Sondag, Joan Hoppe-Bauer, and Lois Himpel. Not only have these three talented individuals alleviated the administrative burdens that accompany a large laboratory, but they are also excellent microbiologists who taught me more than I could ever remember. Finally, I thank my many professional colleagues whose innovative ideas are encompassed in this *Pocket Guide.*

Other key individuals helped bring my ideas and words to a successful conclusion. They include my secretaries, Amy Hall and Jenny Adams, who tolerated unforgiving deadlines; Ann Niles, who helped with editing; Patrick Fitzgerald, director of ASM Press, who gave me complete freedom to develop this book; and Susan Birch, ASM Senior Production Editor, who makes working with ASM Press a professionally successful and emotionally satisfying experience.

Taxonomic Classification of Medically Important Microbes

Taxonomy is defined as the classification of organisms into appropriate categories on the basis of genotypic and phenotypic relationships. Taxonomic classifications have historically been determined by readily observable characteristics such as morphology, biochemical properties, and antigenic relationships. Although these relationships can be readily measured, they are at best an imprecise measure of the similarities or differences among populations of organisms. The traditional phenotypic classification of microbes is rapidly being replaced by classification systems based on genetic homology. This approach is technically more precise but frequently does not lend itself to laboratory identification schemes. Confounding the problem of microbial taxonomy is the frequency with which groups of microbes are subdivided or consolidated into new groups with new names. Thus, *Pseudomonas maltophilia* has been changed to *Xanthomonas maltophilia* and then to *Stenotrophomonas maltophilia*. Likewise, we have witnessed *Neisseria catarrhalis* placed first in the genus *Branhamella* and most recently in the genus *Moraxella*. The reader must recognize that classification schemes are fluid and will continue to evolve as our knowledge of microbiology and microbial pathogenesis expands.

This section is intended to serve as a guide for microbial classification. It is subdivided into four general areas: bacteriology, mycology, virology, and parasitology. The bacteriology subsection is subdivided into genotypic and phenotypic classification schemes. Although the genotypic classification scheme is more precise, identification of medically important bacteria is based primarily on phenotypic characteristics. Likewise, identification of fungi is based on their morphologic appearance. This method complicates the classification of fungi, because they can exist in distinct asexual (anamorph) and sexual (teleomorph) stages, and thus an individual fungus can fit into two different categories within the same classification scheme. For this reason, two schemes for classifying fungi are presented: one is based on morphologic appearance, and the other is based on the sites at which mycotic infections may be encountered. Because arthropods frequently function as vectors or reservoirs of diseases, a table that lists the medically important diseases associated with arthropods is included. For additional information about the taxonomic classification of microbes, please consult the *Manual of Clinical Microbiology,* 6th ed. (1995), *Ber-*

gey's Manual of Determinative Bacteriology (1994), The
Prokaryotes (1992), and Larone's Medically Important Fungi:
a Guide to Identification (1995).

Genotypic Classification of Medically Important Bacteria

Division A: firmicutes (gram-positive bacteria)
**Subdivision A1: firmicutes with high G + C content of
DNA (actinomycetes branch)**

Actinomaduraceae
    Actinomadura
    Actinomyces
Arcanobacterium
Bifidobacterium
Corynebacterium
Gardnerella
Micrococcus
Mobiluncus
Mycobacterium
Nocardiaceae
    Gordona
    Nocardia
    Rhodococcus
    Tsukamurella
Propionibacterium
Rothia
Stomatococcus
Streptomycetaceae
    Streptomyces

**Subdivision A2: firmicutes with low G + C content of
DNA (*Clostridium-Bacillus* branch)**

Aerococcus
Bacillus
Clostridium
Enterococcus
Erysipelothrix
Eubacterium
Gemella
Kurthia
Lactobacillus
Lactococcus

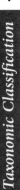

Leuconostoc
Listeria
Mycoplasmatales
   Acholeplasma
   Mycoplasma
   Ureaplasma
Pediococcus
Peptococcus
Peptostreptococcus
Planococcus
Sarcina
Staphylococcus
Streptococcus

Subdivision A3: firmicutes with atypical cell walls (gram-positive eubacteria with gram-negative cell walls)

Butyrivibrio
Megasphaera
Selenomonas
Veillonella

Division B: cyanobacteria

Division C: proteobacteria
Subdivision C1: alpha subclass

Afipia
Bartonella
Brucella
Rickettsiaceae
   Ehrlichia
   Rickettsia

Subdivision C2: beta subclass

Alcaligenaceae
   Alcaligenes
   Bordetella
Burkholderia
Chromobacterium
Comamonadaceae
   Acidovorax
   Comamonas
Leptothrix
Neisseriaceae
   Eikenella
   Kingella
   Neisseria

Ochrobactrum
Oligella
Spirillum

Subdivision C3: gamma subclass
Acinetobacter
Aeromonas
Cardiobacterium
Coxiella
Enterobacteriaceae
    Citrobacter
    Edwardsiella
    Enterobacter
    Escherichia
    Hafnia
    Klebsiella
    Morganella
    Proteus
    Providencia
    Salmonella
    Serratia
    Shigella
    Yersinia
    Many other genera
Legionellaceae
    Fluoribacter
    Legionella
    Tatlockia
Moraxella
    Subgenus: *Branhamella*
Pasteurellaceae
    Actinobacillus
    Haemophilus
    Pasteurella
Plesiomonas
Pseudomonas
Stenotrophomonas
Vibrio

Subdivision C4: delta subclass

Subdivision C5: epsilon subclass
Campylobacter
Helicobacter
Wolinella

Division D: spirochetes
Borrelia
Leptospira
Treponema

Division E: *Chlorobiaceae*

Division F. *Bacteroides* and *Cytophaga* group
Bacteroides
Capnocytophaga
Cytophaga
Flavobacterium
Porphyromonas
Prevotella
Weeksella

Division G: *Chlamydia*

Division H: *Planctomyces* and related bacteria

Division I: *Deinococcaceae* and *Thermus*

Division J: *Chloroflexaceae* and related bacteria

Division K: *Verrucomicrobium*

Division L: *Thermotogales*

Phylogenetically unaffiliated bacteria
Francisella
Fusobacterium
Leptotrichia
Streptobacillus

Phenotypic Classification of Medically Important Bacteria

Aerobic, catalase-positive, gram-positive cocci
Micrococcus
Planococcus
Staphylococcus
Stomatococcus

Aerobic, catalase-negative, gram-positive cocci
Aerococcus
Enterococcus
Gemella
Globicatella
Helcococcus

Lactococcus
Leuconostoc
Pediococcus
Streptococcus
Tetragenococcus
Vagococcus

Anaerobic, gram-positive cocci
Peptococcus
Peptostreptococcus

Aerobic, gram-negative cocci
Branhamella
Neisseria

Anaerobic, gram-negative cocci
Acidaminococcus
Megasphaera
Veillonella

Spore-forming, gram-positive bacilli
Bacillus
Clostridium

Catalase-positive, gram-positive (coryneform) bacilli
Brevibacterium
Cellulomonas
Corynebacterium
Dermabacter
Kurthia
Listeria

Catalase-negative, gram-positive (coryneform) bacilli
Arcanobacterium
Erysipelothrix
Gardnerella

Anaerobic, gram-positive bacilli
Actinomyces
Bifidobacterium
Eubacterium
Lactobacillus
Mobiluncus
Propionibacterium
Rothia

Acid-fast and partially acid-fast actinomycetes (filamentous bacilli)
Gordona
Mycobacterium

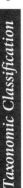

Nocardia
Rhodococcus
Tsukamurella

Non-acid-fast actinomycetes (filamentous bacilli)

Actinomadura
Dermatophilus
Nocardiopsis
Oerskovia
Saccharomonospora
Saccharopolyspora
Streptomyces
Thermoactinomyces

Glucose-fermenting, gram-negative bacilli

Actinobacillus
Capnocytophaga
Cardiobacterium
Chromobacterium
Enterobacteriaceae
   Citrobacter
   Edwardsiella
   Enterobacter
   Escherichia
   Hafnia
   Klebsiella
   Morganella
   Proteus
   Providencia
   Salmonella
   Serratia
   Shigella
   Yersinia
   Many other genera
Haemophilus
Leptotrichia
Pasteurella
Streptobacillus
Suttonella
Vibrionaceae
   Aeromonas
   Plesiomonas
   Vibrio

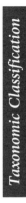

Glucose-oxidizing, gram-negative bacilli

Acidovorax
Acinetobacter
Agrobacterium
Alcaligenes
Brucella
Burkholderia
Chryseomonas
Flavimonas
Flavobacterium
Ochrobactrum
Pseudomonas
Psychrobacter
Roseomonas
Shewanella
Sphingobacterium
Sphingomonas
Stenotrophomonas

Non-glucose-utilizing, gram-negative bacilli

Alcaligenes
Bordetella
Brucella
Burkholderia
Campylobacteraceae
   Arcobacter
   Campylobacter
Comamonadaceae
   Acidovorax
   Comamonas
Eikenella
Flavobacterium
Francisella
Helicobacter
Kingella
Legionella
Moraxella
Oligella
Pseudomonas
Roseomonas
Shewanella
Weeksella
Xanthomonas

Anaerobic, gram-negative bacilli
Bacteroides
Bilophila
Desulfomonas
Fusobacterium
Leptotrichia
Porphyromonas
Prevotella
Selenomonas

Spiral bacilli
Leptospiraceae
Leptonema
Leptospira
Spirochaetaceae
Borrelia
Cristispira
Serpulina
Spirochaeta
Treponema

Cell wall-defective bacteria
Acholeplasmataceae
Acholeplasma
Mycoplasmataceae
Mycoplasma
Ureaplasma

Strict, intracellular bacteria and related organisms
Bartonella
Chlamydiaceae
Chlamydia
Rickettsiales
Coxiella
Ehrlichia
Rickettsia

Taxonomic Classification of Medically Important Fungi

Subdivision: *Zygomycotina*
Class: *Zygomycetes*
Order: *Mucorales*
Genus: *Absidia*
Genus: *Cunninghamella*

Genus: *Mucor*
Genus: *Rhizomucor*
Genus: *Rhizopus*
Genus: *Saksenaea*
Order: *Entomophthorales*
Genus: *Basidiobolus*
Genus: *Conidiobolus*

Subdivision: *Ascomycotina*
Class: *Ascomycetes*
Order: *Endomycetales*
Genus: *Pichia* (teleomorph [sexual] stage of some *Candida* spp.)
Genus: *Saccharomyces*
Order: *Eurotidales*
Family: *Trichocomaceae*
Genus: *Emericella* (*Aspergillus* teleomorph stage)
Genus: *Eurotium* (*Aspergillus* teleomorph stage)
Genus: *Neosartorya* (*Aspergillus* teleomorph stage)
Order: *Onygenales*
Genus: *Ajellomyces* (*Histoplasma* and *Blastomyces* teleomorph stages)
Genus: *Arthroderma* (*Trichophyton* and *Microsporum* teleomorph stages)

Subdivision: *Basidiomycotina*
Class: *Basidiomycetes*
Order: *Agaricales*
Genus: *Agaricus*
Genus: *Amanita*
Order: *Filobasidiales*
Genus: *Filobasidiella* (*Cryptococcus* teleomorph stage)

Subdivision: *Deuteromycotina*
Class: *Blastomycetes*
Order: *Cryptococcales*
Genus: *Candida*
Genus: *Cryptococcus*
Genus: *Hansenula*
Genus: *Malassezia*
Genus: *Rhodotorula*
Genus: *Torulopsis*

Genus: *Trichosporon*
Class: *Hyphomycetes*
  Order: *Moniliales*
    Family: *Moniliaceae*
      Genus: *Acremonium*
      Genus: *Aspergillus*
      Genus: *Chrysosporium*
      Genus: *Coccidioides*
      Genus: *Epidermophyton*
      Genus: *Fusarium*
      Genus: *Paecilomyces*
      Genus: *Paracoccidioides*
      Genus: *Pseudallescheria*
      Genus: *Scedosporium*
      Genus: *Scopulariopsis*
      Genus: *Sporothrix*
    Family: *Dematiaceae*
      Genus: *Alternaria*
      Genus: *Bipolaris*
      Genus: *Cladosporium*
      Genus: *Curvularia*
      Genus: *Exophiala*
      Genus: *Exserohilum*
      Genus: *Fonsecaea*
      Genus: *Phialophora*
      Genus: *Wangiella*
      Genus: *Xylohypha*
Class: *Coelomycetes*
  Order: *Sphaeropsidales*
    Genus: *Phoma*

Morphologic Classification of Medically Important Fungi

Monomorphic yeasts and yeastlike organisms
1. Pseudohyphae with blastoconidia
   Candida spp.
   Hansenula
   Saccharomyces
2. Yeastlike cells only (usually no hyphae or pseudohyphae)
   Cryptococcus
   Hansenula
   Malassezia

  Prototheca
  Rhodotorula
  Saccharomyces
  Sporobolomyces
  Torulopsis
  Ustilago
3. Hyphae and arthroconidia or annelloconidia
  Blastoschizomyces
  Geotrichum
  Trichosporon

Thermally dimorphic fungi
1. *Blastomyces dermatitidis*
2. *Histoplasma capsulatum*
3. *Paracoccidioides brasiliensis*
4. *Penicillium marneffei*
5. *Sporothrix schenckii*

Thermally monomorphic molds
1. White, cream, or light gray surface; nonpigmented reverse
  a. With microconidia or macroconidia
    Acremonium
    Beauveria
    Chrysosporium
    Emmonsia
    Fusarium
    Graphium
    Microsporum
    Pseudallescheria
    Sepedonium
    Stachybotrys
    Trichophyton
    Verticillium
  b. Having sporangia or sporangiola
    Absidia
    Apophysomyces
    Basidiobolus
    Conidiobolus
    Cunninghamella
    Mucor
    Rhizomucor
    Rhizopus
    Saksenaea

      c. Having arthroconidia
  Coccidioides
  Geotrichum
      d. Having only hyphae with chlamydoconidia
  Microsporum
  Trichophyton
2. White, cream, beige, or light gray surface; yellow, orange, or reddish reverse
   Acremonium
   Chaetomium
   Microsporum
   Trichophyton
3. White, cream, beige, or light gray surface; red to purple reverse
   Microsporum
   Penicillium
   Trichophyton
4. White, cream, beige, or light gray surface; brown reverse
   Chaetomium
   Chrysosporium
   Cokeromyces
   Emmonsia
   Madurella
   Microsporum
   Scopulariopsis
   Sporotrichum
   Trichophyton
5. White, cream, beige, or light gray surface; black reverse
   Chaetomium
   Graphium
   Nigrospora
   Phoma
   Pseudallescheria
   Scedosporium
   Trichophyton
6. Tan to brown surface
      a. Having small conidia
  Aspergillus
  Botrytis
  Chrysosporium
  Cladosporium
  Dactylaria
  Emmonsia

      Paecilomyces
      Phialophora
      Pseudallescheria
      Scopulariopsis
      Sporotrichum
      Trichophyton
      Verticillium

  b. Having large conidia or sporangia
      Alternaria
      Apophysomyces
      Basidiobolus
      Bipolaris
      Botrytis
      Cokeromyces
      Conidiobolus
      Curvularia
      Epicoccum
      Epidermophyton
      Fusarium
      Microsporum
      Rhizomucor
      Rhizopus
      Stemphylium
      Trichophyton
      Ulocladium

  c. Having miscellaneous microscopic morphology
      Chaetomium
      Coccidioides
      Madurella
      Phoma
      Ustilago

7. Yellow to orange surface
   Aspergillus
   Chrysosporium
   Epicoccum
   Epidermophyton
   Microsporum
   Monilia
   Penicillium
   Sepedonium
   Sporotrichum
   Trichophyton
   Trichothecium
   Verticillium

8. Pink to violet surface
   Acremonium
   Aspergillus
   Beauveria
   Chrysosporium
   Fusarium
   Gliochadium
   Microsporum
   Monilia
   Paecilomyces
   Sporotrichum
   Trichophyton
   Trichothecium
   Verticillium
9. Green surface; light reverse
   Aspergillus
   Epidermophyton
   Gliocladium
   Penicillium
   Trichoderma
   Verticillium
10. Dark gray or black surface; light reverse
    Aspergillus
    Syncephalastrum
11. Green, dark gray, or black surface; dark reverse
    a. Having small conidia
       Aureobasidium
       Botrytis
       Cladosporium
       Exophiala
       Fonsecaea
       Phaeoannellomyces
       Phialophora
       Pseudallescheria
       Scedosporium
       Wangiella
       Xylohypha
    b. Having large conidia
       Alternaria
       Bipolaris
       Curvularia
       Dactylaria
       Epicoccum

  Helminthosporium
  Nigrospora
  Pithomyces
  Stachybotrys
  Stemphylium
  Ulocladium
 c. Having only hyphae (with or without chlamydoconidia)
  Madurella
  Piedraia
 d. Having large fruiting bodies
  Chaetomium
  Phoma

Taxonomic Classification of Human Viruses

Single-stranded, nonenveloped RNA viruses

Caliciviridae	*Calicivirus*	Human calicivirus, Norwalk virus, Norwalk-like viruses
	Astrovirus	Astrovirus
Picornaviridae	*Enterovirus*	Coxsackievirus groups A and B, echoviruses, enterovirus, poliovirus
	Heparnavirus	Hepatitis A virus
	Cardiovirus	Encephalomyo-carditis virus
	Rhinovirus	Rhinovirus

Single-stranded, enveloped RNA viruses

Arenaviridae	*Arenavirus*	Lymphocytic choriomeningitis virus, Lassa fever virus, Junin virus, Machupo virus, Guanarito virus, Sabia virus

Bunyaviridae	*Bunyavirus*	California encephalitis virus, La Crosse virus
	Phlebovirus	Rift Valley fever virus
	Nairovirus	Crimean-Congo hemorrhagic fever virus
	Hantavirus	Hantaan virus
Coronaviridae	*Coronavirus*	Coronavirus
Filoviridae	*Filovirus*	Ebola virus, Marburg virus
Flaviviridae	*Flavivirus*	Yellow fever virus, dengue virus, St. Louis encephalitis virus
Orthomyxo-viridae	*Influenzavirus*	Influenza virus types A, B, and C
Paramyxoviridae	*Paramyxovirus*	Paramyxovirus, Sendai virus, mumps virus
	Morbillivirus	Measles virus
	Pneumovirus	Respiratory syncytial virus
Retroviridae	HLTV-BLV group	Human T-cell lymphotropic virus types 1 and 2
	Lentivirus	Human immunodeficiency virus types 1 and 2
	Spumavirus	Human foamy virus
Rhabdoviridae	*Lyssavirus*	Rabies virus

| *Togaviridae* | *Alphavirus* | Sindbis virus, Eastern equine encephalitis virus, Western equine encephalitis virus, Venezuelan encephalitis virus, Semliki Forest virus |
| | *Rubivirus* | Rubella virus |

Double-stranded, nonenveloped RNA viruses

Reoviridae	*Orbivirus*	Colorado tick fever virus
	Reovirus	Reovirus
	Rotavirus	Rotavirus

Single-stranded, nonenveloped DNA viruses

| *Parvoviridae* | *Parvovirus* | Parvovirus B19 |
| | *Dependovirus* | Adeno-associated virus |

Double-stranded, nonenveloped DNA viruses

Adenoviridae	*Mastadenovirus*	Adenovirus
Papovaviridae	*Papillomavirus*	Papillomavirus
	Polyomavirus	JC virus, BK virus

Double-stranded, enveloped DNA viruses

Hepadnaviridae	*Hepadnavirus*	Hepatitis B virus
Herpesviridae	*Cytomegalovirus*	Cytomegalovirus
	Lymphocryptovirus	Epstein-Barr virus
	Simplexvirus	Herpes simplex virus
	Varicellovirus	Varicella-zoster virus

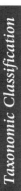

Poxviridae	*Molluscipoxvirus*	Molluscum contagiosum virus
	Orthopoxvirus	Buffalopox virus, cowpox virus, monkeypox virus, vaccinia virus, smallpox virus
	Parapoxvirus	Orf virus

Taxonomic Classification of Medically Important Parasites

Phylum: Sarcomastigophora
Subphylum: Mastigophora (flagellates)
Genus: *Chilomastix*
Genus: *Dientamoeba*
Genus: *Enteromonas*
Genus: *Giardia*
Genus: *Leishmania*
Genus: *Retortamonas*
Genus: *Trichomonas*
Genus: *Trypanosoma*
Subphylum: Sarcodina (amoeba)
Genus: *Acanthamoeba*
Genus: *Blastocystis*
Genus: *Endolimax*
Genus: *Entamoeba*
Genus: *Iodamoeba*
Genus: *Naegleria*

Phylum: Ciliophora (ciliates)
Genus: *Balantidium*

Phylum: Apicomplexa (apicomplexans)
Subclass: Coccidia
Genus: *Cryptosporidium*
Genus: *Cyclospora*
Genus: *Isospora*
Genus: *Plasmodium*
Genus: *Toxoplasma*
Subclass: Piroplasmea
Genus: *Babesia*

Phylum: Microspora (microsporidia)
>> Genus: *Encephalitozoon*
>> Genus: *Enterocytozoon*
>> Genus: *Septata*

Phylum: Platyhelminthes (flatworms)
> Class: Cestoidea (tapeworms)
>> Genus: *Diphyllobothrium*
>> Genus: *Dipylidium*
>> Genus: *Echinococcus*
>> Genus: *Hymenolepis*
>> Genus: *Taenia*
> Class: Trematoda (flukes)
>> Genus: *Clonorchis*
>> Genus: *Fasciola*
>> Genus: *Fasciolopsis*
>> Genus: *Heterophyes*
>> Genus: *Metagonimus*
>> Genus: *Nanophyetus*
>> Genus: *Opisthorchis*
>> Genus: *Paragonimus*
>> Genus: *Schistosoma*

Phylum: Nematoda (roundworms)
> Class: Adenophorea (Aphasmidia)
>> Genus: *Capillaria*
>> Genus: *Trichinella*
>> Genus: *Trichuris*
> Class: Secernentia (Phasmidia)
>> Genus: *Ancylostoma*
>> Genus: *Angiostrongylus*
>> Genus: *Anisakis*
>> Genus: *Ascaris*
>> Genus: *Brugia*
>> Genus: *Dracunculus*
>> Genus: *Enterobius*
>> Genus: *Loa*
>> Genus: *Mansonella*
>> Genus: *Necator*
>> Genus: *Onchocerca*
>> Genus: *Strongyloides*
>> Genus: *Trichostrongylus*
>> Genus: *Wuchereria*

Clinical Classification of Medically Important Parasites

Free-living amebae
Acanthamoeba
Balamuthia
Hartmannella
Naegleria

Intestinal and urogenital protozoa
Amebae
Blastocystis
Endolimax
Entamoeba
Iodamoeba
Ciliate
Balantidium
Coccidia
Cryptosporidium
Cyclospora
Isospora
Sarcocystis
Flagellates
Chilomastix
Dientamoeba
Enteromonas
Giardia
Retortamonas
Trichomonas
Microsporidia
Encephalitozoon
Enterocytozoon
Nosema
Pleistophora
Septata

Blood and tissue protozoa
Babesia
Leishmania
Plasmodium
Toxoplasma
Trypanosoma

Intestinal helminths
Cestodes
Diphyllobothrium (fish tapeworm)
Dipylidium (pumpkin seed tapeworm)
Hymenolepis (dwarf tapeworm)
Taenia (beef and pork tapeworms)
Nematodes
Ancylostoma (Old World hookworm)
Ascaris (roundworm)
Capillaria
Enterobius (pinworm)
Necator (New World hookworm)
Strongyloides (threadworm)
Trichostrongylus
Trichuris (whipworm)
Trematodes
Clonorchis (liver fluke)
Fasciola (liver fluke)
Fasciolopsis (intestinal fluke)
Haplorchis (intestinal fluke)
Heterophyes (intestinal fluke)
Metagonimus (intestinal fluke)
Nanophyetus (intestinal fluke)
Opisthorchis (liver fluke)
Paragonimus (lung fluke)
Pygidiopsis (intestinal fluke)
Schistosoma (blood fluke)
Stellantchasmus (intestinal fluke)

Tissue helminths
Cestodes
Cysticercus (Taenia solium)
Echinococcus
Spirometra
Taenia (coenurosis)
Nematodes
Ancylostoma (dog or cat hookworm)
Angiostrongylus
Anisakis
Brugia (lymphatic filaria)
Capillaria (visceral larva migrans)
Dirofilaria (dog heartworm)
Dracunculus (Guinea worm; subcutaneous tissues)

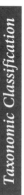

Eustrongylides
Gnathostoma
Loa (eye worm; subcutaneous tissue filaria)
Mansonella (dermal filaria)
Onchocerca (subcutaneous tissue filaria)
Strongyloides
Toxocara (dog or cat ascaris)
Trichinella
Wuchereria (lymphatic filaria)
Trematodes
Clonorchis (liver fluke)
Fasciola (liver fluke)
Paragonimus (lung fluke)
Schistosoma (blood fluke)

Arthropods
Arachnids
Acari (chiggers, mites, ticks)
Araneae (spiders)
Scorpiones (scorpions)
Centipedes
Crustaceans
Copepoda (copepods)
Decapoda (crabs, crayfish)
Millipedes
Insects
Anopleura (sucking lice)
Coleoptera (beetles)
Dictyoptera (cockroaches)
Diptera (flies, midges, mosquitos)
Hemiptera (bedbugs, kissing bugs)
Hymenoptera (ants, bees, wasps)
Lepidoptera (butterflies, caterpillars, moths)
Siphonaptera (fleas)
Tongue worms

Arthropod Vectors of Medically Important Diseases

Arachnida
Acari (ticks)
Dermacentor, Amblyomma
Ehrlichia (ehrlichiosis)

    Francisella tularensis (tularemia)
    Rickettsia rickettsii (Rocky mountain spotted fever)
  Dermacentor
    Coltivirus (Colorado tick fever)
  Ixodes
    Babesis (babesiosis)
    Borrelia burgdorferi (Lyme disease)
    Borrelia spp. (relapsing fever)
  Ornithodoros
    Borrelia spp. (relapsing fever)
Acari (mites)
  Leptotrombidium
    Rickettsia tsutsugamushi (scrub typhus)
  Liponyssoides
    Rickettsia akari (rickettsialpox)

Crustacea
  Copepods (copepods)
    Diphyllobothrium (diphyllobothriasis)
    Dracunculus (Guinea worm disease)
    Gnathostoma (gnathostomiasis)
  Decapods (crabs, crayfish)
    Paragonimus (paragonimiasis)

Insecta
  Anopleura (lice)
    Pediculus
      Bartonella quintana (trench fever)
      Borrelia recurrentis (epidemic relapsing fever)
      Rickettsia prowazekii (epidemic typhus)
  Diptera (mosquitos, flies)
    Aedes
      Flavivirus (dengue, yellow fever)
      Other arboviruses (encephalitis)
    Anopheles
      Arboviruses (encephalitis)
      Brugia malayi (filariasis)
      Plasmodium (malaria)
    Chrysops
      Francisella tularensis (tularemia)
      Loa loa (loiasis)
    Culex
      Arboviruses (encephalitis)

  Brugia spp. (filariasis)
  Wuchereria (filariasis)
 Culicoides
  Mansonella (filariasis)
 Glossina
  Trypanosoma brucei (African sleeping sickness)
 Phlebotomus, Lutzomyia
  Bartonella bacilliformis (bartonellosis)
  Leishmania spp. (leishmaniasis)
  Phlebovirus (sandfly fever)
 Simulium
  Mansonella ozzardi (filariasis)
  Onchocerca volvulus (onchocerciasis)
Hemiptera (bed bugs, kissing bugs)
 Panstrongylus, Rhodnius, Triatoma
  Trypanosoma cruzi (Chagas' disease)
Siphonaptera (fleas)
 Ctenocephalides spp.
  Dipylidium caninum (dog tapeworm disease)
 Nosopsyllus spp.
  Rickettsia typhi (murine typhus)
 Xenopsylla spp.
  Rickettsia typhi (murine typhus)
  Yersinia pestis (plague)

Indigenous and Pathogenic Microbes of Humans

Humans are exposed to microbes at birth, and this exposure leads to one of three nonexclusive interrelationships: transient carriage, persistent colonization, or pathogenic interaction. Most organisms are unable to become established on the skin or mucosal surfaces and are considered insignificant findings when they are recovered in clinical specimens. Examples include many of the nonfermentative gram-negative bacilli and molds that colonize soil, vegetation, water, and food products.

Other organisms are able to establish long-term residency on or in the human body. The successes of these interactions are influenced by complex microbial and host factors (e.g., favorable environment [pH, atmosphere, available nutrients]; ability to adhere to surfaces; resistance to bacteriocins, antibiotics, and phagocytic cells). These microbes generally exist in symbiotic relationships with their human hosts and produce disease only when they invade normally sterile body sites such as tissues and body fluids. Tables 2.1 through 2.3 list the organisms most commonly recovered from the body surfaces of healthy individuals. These tables are intended to provide guidelines for interpreting cultured specimens. The quantitative and qualitative presence of specific microbes, including the indigenous flora in hospitalized patients which can change dramatically, varies with the individual host. Data for viruses are not presented because replication of viruses is generally associated with host tissue destruction or an immunologic response (although this response can range from a clinically asymptomatic infection to host death).

Most diseases in humans are caused by infections with endogenous bacteria and yeasts or by exposure to opportunistic molds, parasites, and viruses. However, some interactions between microbes and humans commonly lead to disease. Examples of these highly virulent pathogenic microbes are summarized in Table 2.4, which is not intended to be an exhaustive list of all exogenous pathogens. For additional information about indigenous and pathogenic microbes, please consult the *Manual of Clinical Microbiology*, 6th ed. (1995), *The Prokaryotes* (1992), Kwon-Chung and Bennett's *Medical Mycology* (1992), Garcia and Bruckner's *Diagnostic Medical Parasitology* (1993), or Mandell, Bennett, and Dolin's *Principles and Practice of Infectious Diseases* (1995).

Table 2.1 Human indigenous flora: bacteria

Organism	Incidence of carriage in[a]:			
	Resp tract	GI tract	GU tract	Skin, ear, and eye
Acholeplasma laidlawii	1+	0	0	0
Acidaminococcus fermentans	1+	0	0	0
Acinetobacter spp.	2+	1+	1+	2+
Actinobacillus spp.	2+	0	0	0
Actinomyces spp.	3+	1+	1+	0
Aerococcus viridans	0	0	0	1+
Aeromonas spp.	0	1+	0	0
Anaerorhabdus furcosus	0	1+	0	0
Arcanobacterium haemolyticum	1+	0	0	0
Bacillus spp.	0	1+	0	1+
Bacteroides fragilis group	1+	3+	1+	0
Bacteroides, other species	1+	2+	1+	0
Bifidobacterium spp.	1+	3+	2+	0
Bilophila wadsworthia	1+	2+	1+	0
Brachyspira aalborgii	0	1+	0	0
Brevibacterium epidermidis	0	0	0	1+

(continued)

Microbes of Humans

Microbes of Humans

Table 2.1 Human indigenous flora: bacteria *(continued)*

Organism	Incidence of carriage in[a]:			
	Resp tract	GI tract	GU tract	Skin, ear, and eye
Burkholderia cepacia	1+	0	0	1+
Butyrivibrio spp.	0	2+	0	0
Campylobacter spp.	2+	1+	0	0
Capnocytophaga spp.	2+	0	1+	0
Cardiobacterium hominis	2+	2+	1+	0
Citrobacter spp.	0	2+	0	0
Clostridium difficile	0	1+	0	0
Clostridium perfringens	0	2+	1+	1+
Clostridium, other species	0	1+	1+	0
Corynebacterium spp.	3+	1+	2+	3+
Dermabacter hominis	0	0	0	1+
Desulfomonas pigra	0	1+	0	0
Desulfovibrio spp.	0	1+	0	0
Eikenella corrodens	2+	1+	1+	0
Enterobacter spp.	1+	2+	0	0
Enterococcus faecalis	0	3+	1+	0
Enterococcus faecium	0	3+	1+	0

Enterococcus, other species	0	1+	1+	0
Escherichia coli	0	3+	1+	0
Eubacterium spp.	2+	3+	1+	0
Flavobacterium meningosepticum	1+	0	0	0
Fusobacterium spp.	3+	1+	0	0
Gardnerella vaginalis	0	0	2+	0
Gemella haemolysans	1+	0	0	0
Gemella morbillorum	1+	1+	0	0
Haemophilus influenzae	3+	1+	1+	0
Haemophilus, other species	3+	1+	1+	0
Hafnia alvei	1+	1+	0	0
Helicobacter pylori	1+	2+	0	0
Kingella denitrificans	1+	0	0	0
Kingella kingae	1+	0	0	0
Klebsiella spp.	1+	2+	0	0
Lactobacillus spp.	1+	3+	3+	0
Leptotrichia buccalis	2+	1+	1+	0
Listeria monocytogenes	0	1+	0	0
Megasphaera elsdenii	1+	0	0	0
Micrococcus spp.	1+	0	0	1+

(continued)

Microbes of Humans

Microbes of Humans

Table 2.1 Human indigenous flora: bacteria *(continued)*

Organism	Resp tract	GI tract	GU tract	Skin, ear, and eye
		Incidence of carriage in[a]:		
Miksuokella multiacidus	0	1+	0	0
Mobiluncus spp.	0	1+	1+	0
Moraxella catarrhalis	2+	0	0	0
Moraxella, other species	1+	0	0	0
Morganella morganii	0	1+	0	0
Mycoplasma spp.	3+	0	3+	0
Neisseria meningitidis	2+	0	1+	0
Neisseria, other species (not gonococcal)	3+	1+	1+	0
Pasteurella multocida	1+	0	0	0
Peptostreptococcus spp.	3+	3+	3+	2+
Porphyromonas spp.	2+	2+	3+	0
Prevotella spp.	3+	2+	3+	0
Propionibacterium spp.	2+	0	1+	3+
Proteus spp.	0	1+	1+	0
Providencia spp.	0	1+	1+	0
Pseudomonas aeruginosa	2+	1+	0	0
Pseudomonas, other species	0	1+	0	0
Rothia dentocariosa	1+	0	0	0

Organism				
Ruminococcus spp.	0	2+	0	0
Selenomonas spp.	2+	1+	0	0
Serpulina spp.	0	1+	0	0
Staphylococcus aureus	3+	1+	1+	1+
Staphylococcus spp., coagulase negative	2+	1+	1+	3+
Stomatococcus mucilaginosus	2+	0	0	0
Streptococcus pneumoniae	2+	0	0	0
Streptococcus pyogenes	2+	0	0	1+
Streptococcus spp., other beta-hemolytic species	2+	1+	1+	0
Streptococcus species viridans group	3+	1+	1+	0
Succinivibrio dextrinosolvens	0	2+	0	0
Tissierella praeacuta	0	1+	0	0
Treponema spp.	3+	2+	2+	1+
Turicella otitidis	0	0	0	1+
Ureaplasma urealyticum	0	0	1+	0
Veillonella spp.	3+	2+	1+	0
Weeksella virosa	0	0	1+	0

[a] Resp, respiratory; GI, gastrointestinal; GU, genitourinary; 3+, commonly present; 2+, frequently isolated; 1+, rarely isolated; 0, not typically isolated.

Microbes of Humans

Microbes of Humans

Table 2.2 Human indigenous flora: fungi

Organism	Incidence of carriage in[a]:			
	Resp tract	GI tract	GU tract	Skin, ear, and eye
Yeasts				
Blastoschizomyces capitatus	0	0	0	1+
Candida albicans	3+	3+	2+	1+
Candida guilliermondii	1+	1+	1+	0
Candida kefyr	1+	1+	1+	0
Candida krusei	1+	1+	1+	0
Candida parapsilosis	2+	2+	0	0
Candida tropicalis	2+	2+	1+	0
Cryptococcus albidus	1+	0	0	0
Malassezia furfur	0	0	0	3+
Malassezia sympodialis	0	0	0	1+
Torulopsis glabrata	2+	2+	2+	0
Rhodotorula spp.	0	0	0	1+
Pneumocystis carinii	1+	0	0	0

Anthropophilic dermatophytes			
Epidermophyton floccosum	0	0	1+
Microsporum audouinii	0	0	1+
Microsporum ferrugineum	0	0	1+
Trichophyton concentricum	0	0	1+
Trichophyton gourvilii	0	0	1+
Trichophyton kanei	0	0	1+
Trichophyton megninii	0	0	1+
Trichophyton mentagrophytes	0	0	1+
Trichophyton raubitschekii	0	0	1+
Trichophyton rubrum	0	0	1+
Trichophyton schoenleinii	0	0	1+
Trichophyton soudanense	0	0	1+
Trichophyton tonsurans	0	0	1+
Trichophyton violaceum	0	0	1+
Trichophyton yaoundei	0	0	1+

[a] Resp, respiratory; GI, gastrointestinal; GU, genitourinary; 3+, commonly present; 2+, frequently isolated; 1+, rarely isolated; 0, not typically isolated.

Table 2.3 Human indigenous flora: protozoa

Organism	Incidence of carriage in[a]:			
	Resp tract	GI tract	GU tract	Skin, ear, and eye
Blastocystis hominis	0	×	0	0
Chilomastix mesnili	0	×	0	0
Endolimax nana	0	×	0	0
Entamoeba coli	0	×	0	0
Entamoeba gingivalis	×	0	0	0
Entamoeba hartmanni	0	×	0	0
Entamoeba polecki	0	×	0	0
Enteromonas hominis	0	×	0	0
Iodamoeba butschlii	0	×	0	0
Retortamonas intestinalis	0	×	0	0
Trichomonas hominis	0	×	0	0
Trichomonas tenax	×	0	0	0

[a] Resp, respiratory; GI, gastrointestinal; GU, genitourinary; 0, parasite absent from this site; ×, parasite can be part of normal flora.

Microbes of Humans

Table 2.4 Pathogenic microbes of humans[a]

Type of organism	Species	
Bacteria	*Bacillus anthracis* *Bordetella parapertussis* *Bordetella pertussis* *Borrelia* spp. *Brucella* spp. *Burkholderia pseudomallei* *Campylobacter coli* *Campylobacter fetus* *Campylobacter jejuni* *Chlamydia* spp. *Corynebacterium diphtheriae* *Coxiella burnetii* *Ehrlichia* spp. *Erysipelothrix rhusiopathiae*	*Francisella tularensis* *Haemophilus ducreyi* *Legionella* spp. *Listeria monocytogenes* *Mycobacterium leprae* *Mycobacterium tuberculosis* complex *Mycoplasma pneumoniae* *Neisseria gonorrhoeae* *Nocardia* spp. *Rickettsia* spp. *Salmonella* spp. *Shigella* spp. *Streptobacillus moniliformis* *Yersinia pestis*
Fungi	*Blastomyces dermatitidis* *Coccidioides immitis* *Cryptococcus neoformans* *Histoplasma capsulatum*	*Paracoccidioides brasiliensis* *Penicillium marneffei* *Pneumocystis carinii*
Viruses	*Arenavirus* group BK virus *Bunyaviridae* group Ebola virus Hepatitis viruses Influenza virus JC virus Marburg virus	Molluscum contagiosum virus Mumps virus Rabies virus *Retroviridae* group Rubella virus
Parasites	*Babesia microti* *Cryptosporidium parvum* *Leishmania* spp. *Plasmodium* spp.	*Toxoplasma gondii* *Trypanosoma* spp. Most intestinal and tissue helminths

[a] Isolation of these microbes is almost always associated with clinically significant human disease.

Microbes of Humans

Specimen Collection and Transport

Precise, sophisticated microbiologic examination of specimens is worthless unless the appropriate specimen is collected and carefully transported to the laboratory. The following section provides guidelines for specimen collection and transport for detection of commonly encountered bacteria, fungi, viruses, and parasites. For additional information, please consult the *Manual of Clinical Microbiology* (6th ed.), *Clinical Microbiology Procedures Handbook,* and J. M. Miller's *A Guide to Specimen Management in Clinical Microbiology* (1996).

Bacteriology

Aerobic, Gram-Positive Cocci

Streptococcus pneumoniae. S. pneumoniae is relatively labile, undergoing spontaneous autolysis and cell death if the specimen is stored in the refrigerator or if culture is delayed.

Other Gram-Positive Cocci. No special precautions are required. Most gram-positive cocci are resistant to desiccation and temperature changes.

Anaerobic, Gram-Positive Cocci

***Peptostreptococcus* spp.** Some *Peptostreptococcus* species are extremely oxygen sensitive; therefore, place the specimens into an appropriate anaerobic container immediately after collection, and maintain them in a moist, anaerobic environment until processing.

Aerobic, Gram-Negative Cocci

***Neisseria* spp.** Neisseriae are extremely labile. Keep specimens moist and under ambient atmosphere (do not refrigerate). Avoid extremes of heat and cold. Ideally, specimens for the recovery of *Neisseria gonorrhoeae* should be inoculated directly onto isolation media at the time of collection. Prewarm the media, and hold the inoculated plates in a carbon dioxide atmosphere during transport to the laboratory. Collect urethral specimens at least 1 h after urination. If urine is processed for *N. gonorrhoeae,* concentrate the urine by centrifugation before processing it. Neisseriae are inhibited by sodium polyanethol sulfonate (SPS), so blood samples should be processed in SPS-free media, in media containing gelatin, or by the lysis-centrifugation system.

Anaerobic, Gram-Negative Cocci

Observe normal precautions for handling anaerobic specimens.

Aerobic, Gram-Positive Bacilli

***Gardnerella* spp.** *Gardnerella* spp. are inhibited by SPS, so blood samples should be processed in SPS-free media, in media containing gelatin, or by the lysis-centrifugation system.

***Listeria* spp.** Listeriae are able to survive and grow at 4°C, while most other bacteria will not survive at this temperature. Specimens can be stored at 4°C to enrich for *Listeria* spp.

Anaerobic, Gram-Positive Bacilli

Observe normal precautions for handling anaerobic specimens.

***Actinomyces* spp.** If sulfur granules are present in drainage material, collect the granules with a sterile loop or forceps, transfer them to a glass slide, and gently crush them. The specimen can be Gram stained and examined under low-power magnification for the presence of filamentous bacilli. Granules should also be crushed and inoculated onto the appropriate culture media.

***Clostridium* spp.** Culture of most *Clostridium* species is relatively easy if spores are present. However, some species (e.g., *Clostridium difficile, C. tetani,* and *C. botulinum*) may be difficult to isolate and will require use of meticulous anaerobic techniques. Refer to the guidelines for selection of specimens for the diagnosis of botulism and *C. perfringens* food-borne diseases. Stool specimens for *C. difficile* cytotoxicity assays can be maintained at 4°C for 3 days or at −70°C for longer periods. Do not store the specimen at −20°C.

Actinomycetes

***Mycobacterium* spp.** Refrigerate specimens (to prevent overgrowth of contaminants) if prolonged transit delays are anticipated. Avoid 24-h collections of respiratory secretions or urine (to avoid overgrowth of contaminants). Neutralize gastric aspirates with sodium carbonate if processing delays in excess of 4 h are anticipated. A minimum of 1 g of tissue is required for adequate processing. Collect blood in a lysis-centrifugation tube, BACTEC 13A bottle, or vacuum tube with SPS or heparin (do not use EDTA as an anticoagulant).

***Nocardia* spp.** Avoid refrigerating specimens for *Nocardia* isolation because some species rapidly lose viability at cold temperatures.

Other Actinomycetes. Collect sulfur granules if present, and process them as described above.

Aerobic, Gram-Negative Bacilli

***Aeromonas* spp.** Process stool specimens for the isolation of *Aeromonas* spp. promptly, or transport them in Cary-Blair medium.

***Bordetella* spp.** Use nasopharyngeal aspirates or swabs (but not throat swabs) for the recovery of *Bordetella pertussis* and *B. parapertussis*. Use Dacron or calcium alginate swabs (not cotton). Inoculate specimens directly onto culture media, or rapidly transport them to the laboratory in 1% casein hydrolysate or in Amies transport medium. If prolonged delays are anticipated before processing, inoculate the specimen into Regan-Lowe semisolid medium.

***Brucella* spp.** No special transport conditions are required other than extreme care in handling the highly infectious specimen.

***Campylobacter* spp.** Process freshly passed stool specimens (rectal swabs can be processed but are not recommended) within 1 h, or transfer the specimen to Cary-Blair medium. Specimens can be stored at 4°C.

***Enterobacteriaceae* (Intestinal Pathogens: *Salmonella* and *Shigella* spp., Selected Strains of *Escherichia coli*, *Yersinia enterocolitica*).** Collect freshly passed stool specimens (not rectal swabs) for recovery of *Enterobacteriaceae* within the first 2 to 3 days of clinical disease. Process specimens within 1 h, or place them in transport medium. Cary-Blair is probably the best overall medium, but others (e.g., Stuart's, Amies, buffered glycerol saline) can be used.

***Francisella* spp.** No special transport conditions are required other than extreme care in handling the highly infectious specimen.

***Helicobacter* spp.** Cimetidine and benzocaine inhibit the growth of these organisms and should be avoided (lidocaine is acceptable). Collect multiple biopsy specimens from the gastric antrum and corpus, and inoculate the specimens directly into sterile saline or Stuart's transport medium. *Helicobacter* spp. are extremely susceptible to drying.

***Legionella* spp.** No special precautions are required for clinical specimens. Collect at least 1 liter of water for processing, and add 0.5 ml of 0.1 N sodium thiosulfate to each liter of chlorinated water. Specimens from faucets and showerheads can be collected with a moist swab and transferred to 3 to 5 ml of water from the receptacle.

***Plesiomonas* spp.**   Refer to *Aeromonas* spp.

***Vibrio* spp.**   Because *Vibrio* strains are susceptible to drying, transport medium is essential if a delay in processing the stool specimens is anticipated. Use of Cary-Blair medium is recommended, and alkaline-peptone water is acceptable if the specimen is processed within 6 to 8 h.

Anaerobic, Gram-Negative Bacilli

Observe normal precautions for handling anaerobic specimens.

Spiral Bacilli

***Borrelia* spp.**   Culturing organisms in the genus *Borrelia* is not commonly attempted. Wright- or Giemsa-stained blood smears can be used to detect borreliae responsible for relapsing fever.

***Leptospira* spp.**   Collect blood and cerebrospinal fluid (CSF) specimens during the first 10 days of illness; collect urine specimens after the first week of illness. Collect blood in tubes with heparin or sodium oxalate but not citrate solutions. Blood and CSF specimens can be stored at 5 to 20°C for up to 1 week before processing, although prompt processing is optimal. Culture urine promptly, or dilute it 1:10 in 1% bovine serum albumin (BSA). Leptospires die rapidly in acidic urine.

***Treponema* spp.**   Diagnosis of syphilis is based on observation of the spirochetes by dark-field microscopy (the organisms are too thin to be detected by bright-field microscopy) or positive serologic tests. Serous fluid free of erythrocytes and tissue debris can be collected on a glass slide and covered with a coverslip. The specimen must be examined within 20 min to detect motile bacteria. The organism will die rapidly when exposed to oxygen, heat, nonphysiologic pH, and desiccation.

Cell Wall-Defective Bacteria

Mycoplasmas.   Throat swabs are as good as expectorated sputum for culturing mycoplasmas. Immediately transfer swabs into transport medium (e.g., nutrient broth with horse serum, double-strength chlamydial sucrose-phosphate transport medium [2SP]). These specimens can be stored at 4°C for 3 days or frozen at −70°C for longer periods.

Ureaplasmas. Urethral swabs or voided urine can be collected for processing. Avoid contact with antiseptics, analgesics, or lubricants. Specimens can be transported and stored as mycoplasmas are.

Intracellular Bacteria and Related Organisms

Chlamydia spp. Chlamydial specimens for culture must include infected cells and not be limited to purulent discharge. Collect specimens by vigorously swabbing or scraping the involved surface (e.g., cervix) and transfer the specimen to 2SP. Cotton, Dacron, and alginate swabs are generally acceptable, although toxicity has been reported with each. Avoid using swabs with wooden shafts. Urine can be used for nonculture procedures (e.g., molecular diagnosis of infections) but is unacceptable for culture because of its toxicity to cell lines.

Ehrlichia spp. Diagnosis is typically made by microscopy, serology, or molecular diagnostic techniques; culture is not normally performed. Anticoagulated blood (use EDTA) can be used for these tests. Heparin can interfere with PCR testing and should be avoided.

Rickettsia spp. See *Ehrlichia* spp.

Mycology

Dermatophytes (*Epidermophyton, Microsporum,* and *Trichophyton* spp.)

Collect infected hairs with sterile forceps (guided by the use of a Wood's lamp if the suspected dermatophyte is fluorescent). Endothrix fungi may require the use of sterile scalpel to collect the hair root. Sample skin lesions at the active border of the lesion, using a sterile scalpel to collect the sample. Disinfect nails with alcohol before the sample is collected by clipping or scraping. Do not place hair, skin, or nail samples in closed tubes. The high humidity fosters overgrowth of contaminating bacteria.

Dimorphic Fungi (*Blastomyces, Coccidioides, Histoplasma, Paracoccidioides,* and *Sporothrix* spp.)

Process specimens (e.g., respiratory, wound aspirates) promptly to avoid overgrowth of contaminating bacteria. Do not use swabs, because these organisms are susceptible to desiccation. *Histoplasma capsulatum* can be recovered in blood cultures, particularly from patients with AIDS and other immunosuppressive diseases. Collect blood specimens by using a lysis-centrifugation system.

Eumycotic Mycetoma Agents (*Acremonium, Curvularia, Corynespora, Cylindrocarpon, Emericella, Exophiala, Fusarium, Leptosphaeria, Madurella, Neotestudina, Plenodomus, Polycytella, Pseudallescheria, Pseudochaetosphaeronema,* and *Pyrenochaeta* spp.)

Examine pus, exudate, or biopsy material for the presence of granules consisting of the eumycotic agents and matrix material. Wash the granules with saline containing antibiotics (e.g., penicillin and streptomycin), and then culture them. Organisms can be visualized by examining crushed granules microscopically.

Moniliaceous Fungi

Process specimens promptly to avoid overgrowth of contaminating bacteria. Do not use swabs, because these organisms are susceptible to desiccation. *Pseudallescheria boydii* and *Fusarium* spp. are among the few filamentous fungi that can be recovered in blood cultures. Collect blood specimens for these fungi by using a lysis-centrifugation system.

Pneumocystis spp.

Respiratory specimens should be limited to induced sputa or bronchoscopy specimens. Patients can only rarely expectorate sputum, and throat washings are insensitive. Collect first morning specimens when possible. A 24-h collection is unacceptable. The presence of oral contamination, signified by squamous epithelial cells, does not invalidate examination of the specimen.

Yeasts

Yeasts are relatively easy to isolate from clinical specimens, although overgrowth of contaminating bacteria should be avoided. Because yeasts are a relatively common isolate from blood specimens, select culture systems that optimize the recovery of these organisms. The lysis-centrifugation system and biphasic culture systems are the most reliable methods for isolating yeasts from blood samples.

Virology

GENERAL GUIDELINES

1. Transport specimens collected on swabs in a moist environment, such as viral transport medium (e.g., viral Culturette

Specimen Collection

system), 2SP, or other suitable liquid medium. Dried specimens are unacceptable because many viruses, particularly enveloped viruses, will not survive drying.

2. Avoid calcium alginate fiber swabs, charcoal-impregnated swabs, and swabs with wooden shafts, because viral infectivity may be inactivated or toxicity to cell lines may occur.

3. Specimens collected by washings (e.g., nasopharyngeal specimens) may be supplemented with gelatin or BSA to stabilize the viruses.

4. Collect vesicle fluids and skin scrapings without using skin disinfectants, because disinfectants may contaminate the specimen and inactivate the viruses.

5. Collect blood specimens using citrate or heparin as an anticoagulant. If the specimen is to be processed for PCR tests, avoid heparin, because it will bind DNA and cause false-negative reactions.

6. Store specimens for viral culture either at 4 to 8°C or frozen at -70°C. Do not store specimens at -20°C. Specimens can be diluted with an equal volume of 2SP before freezing to protect labile viruses; however, use of other cryopreservatives such as sorbitol or glycerin is not recommended. Ideally, avoid using diluents and freezing, because they reduce the number of infectious viruses inoculated onto cell cultures.

7. Many viruses (e.g., arenaviruses, hantaviruses, filoviruses, lentiviruses, and lyssaviruses) are extremely dangerous. Exercise appropriate care when handling these specimens and other infectious viruses.

SPECIFIC GUIDELINES

Single-Stranded, Nonenveloped RNA Viruses

Astrovirus and Calicivirus. Astroviruses can be grown in cell culture, but this has not been accomplished for the calicivirus group. Caliciviruses, such as Norwalk virus, can be detected by PCR and electron microscopy. Collect fecal specimens for the isolation of astroviruses within the first 2 days of clinical illness. Viruses are relatively stable and will maintain infectivity for up to 1 week at 4°C or for more extended periods at -70°C. Preservatives or transport media are generally not required.

Enterovirus. Infections with enteroviruses are confirmed by culture or animal inoculations. Viruses can be recovered from serum, whole blood, CSF, urine, throat washings, and fecal specimens (depending on the clinical disease). Maintain specimens in a moist environment, in which the viruses are very stable. Virus infectivity can be maintained for weeks at 4°C and for years at −70°C. Infectivity decreases more rapidly when specimens are stored at ambient temperatures.

Heparnavirus. Isolation of hepatitis A virus (HAV) in culture is extremely difficult and is rarely done. Infections with HAV are generally confirmed by serologic tests or antigen detection assays. HAV antigen can be detected in fecal specimens 2 weeks before and several days after onset of illness. Fecal specimens can be diluted in buffered saline with 0.02% sodium azide and stored for up to 4 months at 4°C or for more prolonged periods at −70°C.

Rhinovirus. Rhinoviral infections are confirmed by isolation of rhinoviruses in cell cultures. The highest concentrations of viruses occur in nasal secretions during the first 1 to 2 days of illness. Nasal washings are the preferred specimen. If swabs are collected, store them in an appropriate transport medium. Specimens can be stored at 4°C for 1 day or at −70°C for longer periods.

Single-Stranded, Enveloped RNA Viruses

Arbovirus. Few laboratories attempt to isolate arboviruses. Most infections are confirmed by serologic assays. Samples for culture should be maintained at 4°C for 1 to 2 days or frozen at −70°C.

Arenavirus and Filovirus. Infection with viruses from these groups is confirmed by viral isolation in culture (rarely performed except by experienced investigators), microscopy, or serologic testing. Lymphocytic choriomeningitis virus may be recovered from blood and CSF within the first week of disease but rarely from throat washings or urine. Lassa virus can be isolated from acute-phase sera and throat washings but is less frequently isolated from urine. Junin virus can be isolated from sera and throat washings during the first 10 days of clinical disease. For each virus, serum or heparinized blood is better than whole blood. Freeze specimens on dry ice or in liquid nitrogen. Throat washings and urine can be mixed with a buffered diluent containing serum proteins to stabilize viral infectivity during freezing.

Influenza Virus. Laboratory diagnosis of influenza virus infections includes isolation of viruses in cell culture, immunologic detection of viral antigens, detection of viral nucleic acids by hybridization or PCR tests, and serology. Collect specimens (e.g., nasopharyngeal washings and aspirates) for culture within the first 72 h of disease, and transport them to the laboratory in the appropriate medium (e.g., cell culture medium, tryptose phosphate broth, or veal infusion broth). Stabilize these specimens with protein (e.g., BSA or gelatin) and antibiotics. Specimens can be stored at 4°C for up to 4 days or at −70°C for more prolonged periods.

Lentivirus.   Human immunodeficiency virus infections are commonly diagnosed by serologic tests. Blood treated with heparin or EDTA can be used for culture, but avoid heparin if the specimen is to be tested by PCR.

Measles Virus.   Culture of measles virus is rarely attempted, because viral recovery is generally low. Viral antigens can be detected in infected cells by direct immunofluorescence or immunoassay. Viral antibodies can also be detected. Culture or direct antigen detection can be attempted with nasopharyngeal aspirates. Specimens can be stored at 4°C but should not be frozen.

Mumps Virus.   The laboratory diagnosis of mumps infection is by viral isolation or serologic testing. Direct immunofluorescence testing of virus-infected cells has been successful with other paramyxoviruses but has not been systematically studied with mumps virus. Virus can be isolated in saliva for 9 days before and up to 8 days after the onset of symptoms. Virus can be isolated in urine for 2 weeks after the onset of symptoms. The highest yield is early in the course of disease.

Parainfluenza Virus.   Infections with parainfluenza viruses are diagnosed by viral isolation in cell cultures, direct detection of viral antigens in infected cells, PCR detection of viral nucleic acids, or serologic testing. Collect nasopharyngeal washings or nasal swabs, and transport them in the appropriate medium for viral isolation or antigen detection (see Influenza Virus above). Specimens can be held at 4°C or stored for long periods at −70°C.

Rabies Virus.   Brain tissue is the most reliable diagnostic specimen for detecting rabies virus, although viral antigens can be detected in saliva, cutaneous nerves, or other tissues. Maintain the specimen at 4°C for no more than 2 days, or store it on dry ice. Do not store specimens in preservatives.

Respiratory Syncytial Virus.   Laboratory diagnosis of respiratory syncytial virus infections is by viral isolation, direct detection of viral antigens by immunofluorescence or immunoassay, and serology. For the greatest recovery of viruses in infected epithelial cells, collect nasopharyngeal washings and aspirates. Maintain specimens in the appropriate transport medium (see Influenza Virus above) at 4°C. Infectivity is lost rapidly at room temperature or after freezing. This loss may be ameliorated by treating the specimen with stabilizers such as sucrose or glycerin.

Rubella Virus. Viral cultures for rubella virus are rarely performed except when congenital disease is suspected. Diagnosis of rubella infection or prior exposure to the virus is by serologic testing.

Double-Stranded, Nonenveloped RNA Viruses

Rotavirus. Rotaviruses are difficult to recover in cell cultures, serologic tests are rarely performed, and use of PCR is restricted to research laboratories. Historically, rotavirus infections were diagnosed by electron microscopy. Although this technique is still used in some laboratories, diagnosis is now primarily by antigen detection tests (e.g., immunoassays and latex agglutination with specific antibody preparations). Collect stool specimens during the first 3 to 5 days of illness. Do not use preservatives and transport media. Inhibitors in the preservatives may interfere with antigen detection tests, and antibodies to rotaviruses may be present in the serum of the transport media. Maintain specimens at 4°C until they are assayed.

Single-Stranded, Nonenveloped DNA Viruses

Parvovirus. Infection with parvovirus B19 is determined by serologic assay for immunoglobulin M antibody or detection of virus by counterimmunoelectrophoresis, electron microscopy, immunoassays, or PCR tests. Serum is the specimen used for diagnosis; it should be stored at 4°C before testing.

Double-Stranded, Nonenveloped DNA Viruses

Adenovirus. Diagnosis of adenovirus infections is by culture or serologic testing. The viruses are stable and can be easily recovered from clinically involved sites of infection. Nasopharyngeal swabs or aspirates, conjunctival swabs, rectal swabs, urine, urethral or cervical swabs, and tissues are all appropriate specimens. Collect specimens early in the course of disease, and then maintain them at 4°C until processing.

Papillomavirus. Human papillomaviruses cannot be cultured, so diagnosis of infections is by microscopy or detection

Specimen Collection

of viral DNA. Collect genital specimens with adequate numbers of infected epithelial cells.

Polyomavirus.   Diagnosis of JC virus and BK virus infections is by viral isolation (not routinely performed), antigen detection in tissues (e.g., brain, kidney, or bone marrow), detection of viral DNA by PCR tests, and serology. Urine is the optimal specimen for detection of BK virus. JC virus is most frequently detected in infected brain tissues. Blood can be collected in heparin or citrate (avoid heparin with PCR tests).

Double-Stranded, Enveloped DNA Viruses

Cytomegalovirus.   Infections with cytomegalovirus are demonstrated by isolation of the virus from urine, throat washings, saliva, and buffy coat preparation; direct detection of virus-infected cells by microscopy; or detection of viral DNA by PCR tests. Maintain specimens for culture at 4°C if they cannot be inoculated directly into the culture systems at the time of collection.

Hepadnavirus.   Confirmation of hepatitis B virus infection is by serology or PCR detection of viral DNA. Blood samples for PCR testing can be collected in citrate or EDTA, but avoid heparin. Process samples within 6 h, or store them at −70°C.

Lymphocryptovirus.   Epstein-Barr virus infections are generally confirmed by serology. Although isolation of virus is possible, it is rarely attempted in clinical laboratories. When viral isolation is performed, infected cells are collected by having the patient gargle with 5 to 10 ml of serum-free tissue culture medium or Hanks' balanced salt solution. Fetal bovine serum and antibiotics can be added to stabilize the collected specimen. Under these conditions, the specimen can be stored at 4°C for 2 to 3 days.

Molluscipoxvirus.   Infections with molluscum contagiosum virus are diagnosed by clinical presentation. The virus cannot be isolated in culture, and no serologic test is available.

Orthopoxvirus.   Any suspicion of smallpox infection must be reported to the state health department immediately. Specimens for confirmation of other poxvirus infections should include vesicular fluid with cells from the base of the vesicle, encrusted tops of lesions, and appropriate tissue specimens (e.g., skin, liver, spleen, lung, or kidney). Vesicular fluid can be collected on glass slides or in capillary tubes. Do not store specimens in transport fluid. They can be held at 4°C for a short time or at −70°C for prolonged periods.

Simplexvirus. Infections with herpes simplex viruses can be diagnosed by viral isolation, antigen detection, detection of viral DNA by PCR assays, and serology. Specimens for viral isolation or detection can be aspirated or collected with a swab. Cotton swabs are preferred, because viral infectivity can be reduced on calcium alginate swabs. Use a premoistened swab to absorb vesicle fluid, and then vigorously rub the swab on the base of the lesion to collect infected epithelial cells. The specimen can be directly inoculated into culture media or placed in transport media. Specimens can be maintained at 4°C for up to 2 days.

Varicellovirus. Specimens for isolation of varicella-zoster virus include skin scrapings, vesicular cells, and tissues such as lung. Tissue specimens can also be examined by microscopy or tested by PCR, and blood can be collected for serologic testing. Specimens for viral detection should include cells from the bases of the vesicles, because relatively few viruses will be present in the vesicular fluid. Specimens can be collected on swabs and either inoculated directly into culture media or stored in transport media at 4°C. Do not process crusted lesions.

Parasitology

GENERAL GUIDELINES

1. Mineral oil and barium bismuth can make examination of fecal specimens impossible, because protozoa and eggs are obscured by these preparations. Collect specimens before treatment, or else parasitic examination will have to be delayed for 1 week or more.

2. Antibiotics and antimalarial agents can interfere with examination of fecal specimens for protozoa by reducing the numbers of parasites for up to 2 weeks.

3. Trophozoites die rapidly in collected stool specimens. If detection of motility is attempted, then the specimen must be examined within 30 to 60 min of collection. If this cannot be done, then use of preservatives is recommended (see Table 3.3).

SPECIFIC GUIDELINES

Free-Living Amebae

The laboratory diagnosis of infections with free-living amebae can be accomplished by isolation of the organisms in culture, direct examination of clinical material, or serologic testing (primarily used to confirm infection and not to make a diagnosis or to guide therapy). Specimens for isolation include CSF, corneal biopsy samples and scrapings, and brain or lung tissue, depending on the patient's clinical presentation. Collect specimens aseptically and maintain them at room temperature until processing. Storage at 4°C for less than 24 h can be done but should be avoided, because there is a significant loss of viable organisms. Preserve tissues for histological examination in 10% neutral buffered formalin until they are examined histologically.

Intestinal and Urogenital Protozoa

Amebae. The laboratory identification of amebic infections is most commonly accomplished by the microscopic detection of organisms in stool specimens. *Entamoeba histolytica* antigens can also be detected by immunoassays, and antibody production in response to extraintestinal disease is measured by serologic tests. Amebic trophozoites will not survive in unpreserved stool specimens, so specimens should be examined within 30 to 60 min of evacuation. Use of preservatives is required if specimen examination is delayed. Extraintestinal infections are generally confirmed by serologic testing although detection of amebae in abscess material or liver biopsy samples is possible.

Ciliates. Infection with *Balantidium* spp. is confirmed by the microscopic examination of voided stool specimens.

Coccidia. Detection of coccidia in stool specimens is difficult because the coccidia are small, do not stain well with traditional parasitic stains (e.g., iodine, trichrome, iron hematoxylin), and are shed intermittently. Examine several stool specimens. *Cryptosporidium* infections can be detected by acid-fast stains, as well as immunofluorescence and enzyme immunoassays that detect antigen in stool specimens.

Flagellates. Infections with *Giardia lamblia* can be detected by the microscopic examination of stool specimens and by enzyme immunoassay or direct fluorescent-antibody assay for *Giardia* antigen. Examine several stool specimens to confirm or exclude infection. Occasionally, the string test must be used to detect trophozoites in duodenal mucus. Duodenal biopsy may also reveal *G. lamblia*. *Trichomonas vaginalis* is responsible for some urogenital infections. Trophozoites can be observed in vaginal or prostatic secretions. Urine can be examined, but it must not be contaminated with fecal material (which can contain nonpathogenic *Trichomonas* spp.). The urine specimens examined must be freshly collected, because the trophozoites deteriorate rapidly. Immunofluorescence and immunoassays for antigen detection have been developed.

Microsporidia. Like coccidia, microsporidia are difficult to detect in stool specimens. Multiple specimens must be examined. Biopsied tissue may also be useful. Electron microscopy is considered the ''gold standard'' for confirming these infections.

Blood and Tissue Protozoa

Babesia **sp.** Diagnosis of babesiosis requires examination of several thick and thin smears of blood, because low-grade parasitemia is common. Serologic tests have been developed, but cross-reactivity with *Plasmodium* spp. has been reported.

Leishmania **spp.** Diagnosis of cutaneous and visceral leishmaniasis is accomplished by detection of amastigotes in clinical specimens or promastigotes in culture. Collect cutaneous specimens after the surface of the lesion has been disinfected with 70% alcohol. Collect samples (scrapings or biopsy specimens) from the margins of active lesions (the centers do not contain organisms). Specimens for the diagnosis of visceral leishmaniasis include spleen tissue (optimal), nasal secretions, tonsillopharyngeal mucosae, lymph node aspirates, liver biopsy samples, bone marrow, and buffy coat preparations. Prepare multiple slides for staining at the time of collection. Collect specimens for culture or animal inoculation aseptically to prevent bacterial contamination. Standardized serologic tests are not commercially available at this time. The leishmanin (Montenegro) skin test has been used, but reactivity is generally delayed until the convalescence stage.

Plasmodium **spp.** Examine multiple blood specimens over a 36-h period, using both thick and thin smears, to confirm the diagnosis of malaria. This is especially important if the patient has been partially treated. Collect blood by finger stick, and treat the blood with either heparin or EDTA (preferred) as an anticoagulant. If blood smears are not prepared within 1 h of specimen collection, the morphology of the infected cells will be adversely affected. Antigen detection and PCR methods have been developed but are not in common use. Serologic testing is not useful for diagnosis but can confirm previous disease.

Specimen Collection

Toxoplasma gondii.   Infections with *T. gondii* are confirmed by detection of the organism in biopsy specimens, buffy coat cells, or CSF or by isolation of the organism from specimens inoculated into tissue culture or laboratory animals. Because asymptomatic carriage of the organism may occur, the most reliable diagnostic tests are detection of tachyzoites in CSF or bronchoalveolar lavage fluid. Serologic testing may also be helpful.

Trypanosomes.   African trypanosomiasis, caused by *Trypanosoma brucei,* is diagnosed by detection of trypomastigotes in blood, lymph node and bone marrow aspirates, and CSF. Collect blood by finger stick or venipuncture with EDTA. Prepare multiple thick and thin smears. Maximum parasitemia occurs during febrile episodes; if the blood is negative, examine lymph node aspirates. Immunoassays have been used to detect antigens in serum and CSF, and antibodies have been detected by serologic tests. American trypanosomiasis, or Chagas' disease, caused by *Trypanosoma cruzi,* is diagnosed by examining thick and thin smears of blood and buffy coat cells and by examining aspirates from chagomas and enlarged lymph nodes and biopsy specimens for amastigotes and trypomastigotes. Culture of blood, aspirates, and tissues can also be performed. Serologic testing can be used to confirm infections.

Intestinal Helminths

Cestodes.   Diagnosis of infections with intestinal cestodes is by detection of eggs or proglottids in fecal specimens.

Nematodes.   Infections with intestinal nematodes are generally confirmed by detection of the characteristic eggs in fecal specimens. The exception to this is strongyloidiasis, in which larvae are found in stool. Because detection of *Strongyloides* spp. may be difficult, examine multiple stool specimens. Special procedures for other nematodes include use of the cellulose tape technique for sampling the anal folds of patients infected with *Enterobius vermicularis.*

Trematodes.   Infections with intestinal trematodes are typically confirmed by detection of eggs in fecal specimens or, in the case of *Paragonimus* spp. and some schistosomes, eggs in sputum and urine specimens, respectively. Intestinal biopsies have been useful for diagnosing some parasitic infestations.

Tissue Helminths

Cestodes.   The diagnosis of infections with cestodes is based on the patient's clinical presentation, the patient's history of specific travel or diet, and laboratory procedures such as serologic reactivity or observation of the characteristic parasitic structures in tissue. Diagnosis of sparganosis, caused by *Spirometra* spp., is confirmed by recovery of the intact worm in the subcutaneous tissue mass or detection by histologic examination of the tissue. The diagnosis of cysticercosis, caused by *Taenia solium,* and coenurosis, produced by larval *Taenia* spp., is established by recovery of cysticerci or histologic demonstration of cysticerci in tissue. Hydatid disease, caused by *Echinococcus* spp., is diagnosed by radiologic demonstration of cysts and serologic testing. Aspiration of fluid containing ''hydatid sand'' is considered hazardous and should not be attempted.

Nematodes. Infections with filarial nematodes are confirmed by detection of microfilariae in blood or skin or detection of the adult worms in tissues. Adult lymphatic filariae (*Wuchereria* and *Brugia* spp.) are present in lymphatic tissues; their microfilariae migrate in the blood. *Wuchereria* microfilariae are nocturnal, and *Brugia* microfilariae are periodic. Adult *Loa loa* worms are found either in subcutaneous tissues or in the conjunctivae (eye worm); the microfilariae migrate in the blood during the daytime. Because relatively few microfilariae are present in blood, diagnosis of filariasis caused by these nematodes generally requires concentration of blood by filtration and examination of thick smears. Thin smears are usually not useful. *Onchocerca* adult worms are in fibrous subcutaneous nodules, and the microfilaria can be detected in skin and occasionally in the cornea and anterior chamber of the eye. Skin snips are obtained by biopsies of the scapular region, iliac crest, and calf. Be careful not to cause bleeding, which may confound diagnosis if blood microfilariae are present. *Mansonella* species can be found in either skin tissues or blood, depending on the species. *Dracunculus* adult worms live in subcutaneous tissues and release larvae after migrating to the skin surface. Diagnosis depends on recovery of adult female worms at the surface of the skin. Diagnosis of trichinosis, caused by *Trichinella spiralis,* is confirmed by demonstrating encapsulated larvae in biopsy samples of skeletal muscle (e.g., deltoid, gastrocnemius) or serologic reactivity. Nematodes associated with larva migrans are recovered by detection of eggs or larva in tissues or serologic reactivity.

Trematodes. Most trematode infections are generally diagnosed by detection of characteristic eggs in fecal specimens. However, adult worms and occasionally eggs can be found in tissues. Identification of the worms and eggs is based on their morphologic characteristics and anatomical locations.

Specimen Collection

Specimen Collection

Table 3.1 General specimen collection and transport guidelines for bacteria and fungi[a]

| Specimen type | Collection | | Time and temp | |
	Guidelines	Device and/or minimum vol	Transport	Storage
Abscess				
Open	Remove surface exudate by wiping with sterile saline or 70% alcohol. Aspirate if possible, or pass swab deep into lesion, and firmly sample lesion's advancing edge.	Swab transport system	≤2 h, RT	≤24 h, RT
Closed	Aspirate abscess wall material with needle and syringe. Aseptically transfer *all* material into anaerobic transport device or vial.	Anaerobic transport system, ≥1 ml	≤2 h, RT	≤24 h, RT
Bite wound	See Abscess.			
Blood culture	For disinfection of culture bottle, apply 70% isopropyl alcohol to rubber stoppers, and wait 1 min. For disinfection of venipuncture site: 1. Cleanse site with 70% alcohol. 2. Swab concentrically, starting at center, with iodine.	Bacteria: blood culture, 2 bottles/set Adult, 20 ml/set Child, 5–10 ml/set Infant, 1–2 ml/set Fungi 1. Biphasic culture	≤2 h, RT	

	3. Allow iodine to dry. 4. *Do not palpate vein.* 5. Collect blood. 6. After venipuncture, remove iodine from skin with alcohol.	or 2. Lysis centrifuge system	
Catheter i.v.	1. Cleanse skin around catheter site with alcohol. 2. Remove catheter aseptically, and clip 5-cm distal tip of catheter directly into sterile tube or cup. 3. Transport directly to microbiology laboratory to prevent drying.	Sterile screw-cap tube or cup	≤15 min, RT ≤24 h, 4°C
Foley	Do *not* culture, since growth represents distal urethral flora.		
Cellulitis	1. Cleanse site by wiping with sterile saline or 70% alcohol. 2. Aspirate area of maximum inflammation with fine needle and syringe.	Capped syringe or sterile tube	≤15 min, RT ≤24 h, 4°C

(continued)

Specimen Collection

Specimen Collection

Table 3.1 General specimen collection and transport guidelines for bacteria and fungi[a] (*continued*)

Specimen type	Collection Guidelines	Device and/or minimum vol	Time and temp Transport	Time and temp Storage
	3. Draw small amount of sterile saline into syringe. 4. Remove needle (with protective device), and cap.			
CSF	1. Disinfect site with iodine. 2. Insert needle with stylet at L3-L4, L4-L5, or L5-S1 interspace. 3. When needle reaches subarachnoid space, remove stylet, and collect 1–2 ml of fluid into each of 3 leakproof tubes.	Sterile screw-cap tube Bacteria, ≥1 ml Fungi, ≥2 ml AFB, ≥2 ml Virus, ≥1 ml	Bacteria: ≤15 min, RT (never refrigerate) Virus: ≤15 min, 4°C (send on ice)	≤2 h, RT ≤72 h, 4°C
Decubitus ulcer	1. Cleanse surface with sterile saline. 2. If biopsy sample is not available, *vigorously* swab base of lesion. 3. Place swab in appropriate transport system.	Swab transport or anaerobic system	≤2 h, RT	≤24 h, RT
Dental culture: gingival, periodontal, periapical, Vincent's stomatitis	1. Carefully cleanse gingival margin and supragingival tooth surface to remove saliva, debris, and plaque.	Anaerobic transport system	≤2 h, RT	≤24 h, RT

	2. Using periodontal scaler, carefully remove subgingival lesion material, and transfer it to anaerobic transport system.		
	3. Prepare smears collected in same fashion.		
Ear			
Inner	Tympanocentesis is reserved for complicated, recurrent, or chronic persistent otitis media.	Sterile tube, swab transport medium, or anaerobic system	≤2 h, RT ≤2 h, RT ≤2 h, RT
	1. For intact ear drum, clean ear canal with soap solution, dry canal, and collect fluid via syringe aspiration technique.		
	2. For ruptured ear drum, collect fluid on flexible-shaft swab via auditory speculum.		
Outer	1. Use moistened swab to remove any debris or crust from ear canal.	Swab transport	≤2 h, RT ≤24 h, 4°C
	2. Obtain sample by firmly rotating swab in outer canal.		

(continued)

Specimen Collection

Specimen Collection

Table 3.1 General specimen collection and transport guidelines for bacteria and fungi[a] *(continued)*

Specimen type	Collection		Time and temp	
	Guidelines	Device and/or minimum vol	Transport	Storage
Eye				
Conjunctival	1. Sample both eyes with separate swabs (premoistened with sterile saline) by rolling swab over each conjunctiva. 2. Inoculate medium at time of collection. 3. Smear swabs onto 2 slides for staining.	Direct culture inoculation	Plates; ≤15 min, RT	≤2 h, RT
Corneal scrapings	1. Obtain conjunctival swab specimens as described above. 2. Instill 2 drops of local anesthetic. 3. Using sterile spatula, scrape ulcers or lesions, and inoculate scraping directly onto medium. 4. Apply remaining material to 2 clean glass slides for staining.	Direct culture inoculation	Plates; ≤15 min, RT	≤2 h, RT

Feces			
Routine culture	Pass directly into clean, dry container. Transport to microbiology laboratory within 1 h of collection, or transfer to enteric transport system.	Sterile, leakproof, wide-mouth container or enteric transport system, ≥2 g	Unpreserved: ≤1 h, RT	≤24 h, 4°C Enteric transport system: ≤48 h, RT
Clostridium difficile	Pass liquid or soft stool directly into clean, dry container. Soft stool is defined as stool that assumes shape of its container.	Sterile, leakproof, wide-mouth container, ≥5 ml	≤1 h, RT	≤24 h, 4°C >24 h, −20°C
Escherichia coli O157:H7	Pass liquid and/or bloody stool into clean, dry container.	Sterile, leakproof, wide-mouth container or enteric transport system, >2 ml	Unpreserved: ≤1 h, RT	≤24 h, 4°C Enteric transport system: ≤48 h, RT
Rectal swab	1. Carefully insert swab ≈1 in. (≈2.5 cm) beyond anal sphincter. 2. Gently rotate swab to sample anal crypts.	Swab transport	≤1 h, RT	≤24 h, RT
Fistulas	See Abscess.			

(continued)

Specimen Collection

Table 3.1 General specimen collection and transport guidelines for bacteria and fungi[a] *(continued)*

| | Collection | | Time and temp | |
| | | | | |
Specimen type	Guidelines	Device and/or minimum vol	Transport	Storage
Fluids: abdominal, ascites, bile, joint, pericardial, peritoneal, pleural, synovial	1. Disinfect overlying skin with iodine. 2. Obtain specimen via percutaneous needle aspiration or surgery. 3. Transport immediately to laboratory. 4. Always submit as much fluid as possible; *never* submit swab dipped in fluid.	Sterile screw-cap tube or anaerobic transport system, ≥1 ml. Specimens for bacterial or fungal culture can be inoculated directly into blood culture bottles.	≤15 min, RT	≤2 h, RT, except pericardial fluid and fungal cultures
Gangrenous tissue	See Abscess.			
Gastric: wash or lavage fluid	Collect in early morning before patients eat and while they are still in bed. 1. Introduce nasogastric tube orally or nasally into stomach. 2. Perform lavage with 25–50 ml of chilled, sterile, distilled water.	Sterile leakproof container	≤15 min, RT, or neutralize within 1 h of collection	≤24 h, 4°C

		Procedure	Transport system	Time/temp
		3. Recover sample, and place in leakproof sterile container.		
		4. Before removing tube, release suction, and clamp tube.		
Genital: female				
Amniotic		1. Aspirate via amniocentesis, cesarean section, or intrauterine catheter.	Anaerobic transport system, ≥1 ml	≤15 min, RT
		2. Transfer fluid to anaerobic transport system.		≤2 h, RT
Bartholin		1. Disinfect skin with iodine.	Anaerobic transport system, ≥1 ml	≤2 h, RT
		2. Aspirate fluid from ducts.		
Cervical		1. Visualize cervix with speculum without lubricant.	Swab transport	≤2 h, RT
		2. Remove mucus and/or secretions from cervix with swab, and discard swab.		
		3. Firmly yet gently, sample endocervical canal with sterile swab.		
Cul-de-sac		Submit aspirate or fluid.	Anaerobic transport system, >1 ml	≤2 h, RT

(continued)

Specimen Collection

Table 3.1 General specimen collection and transport guidelines for bacteria and fungi[a] (*continued*)

| Specimen type | Collection | | Time and temp | |
	Guidelines	Device and/or minimum vol	Transport	Storage
Endometrial	1. Collect transcervical aspirate via telescoping catheter. 2. Transfer entire amount to anaerobic transport system.	Anaerobic transport system, ≥1 ml	≤2 h, RT	≤2 h, RT
Products of conception	1. Submit portion of tissue in sterile container. 2. If obtained by cesarean section, immediately transfer to anaerobic transport system.	Sterile tube or anaerobic transport system	≤2 h, RT	≤2 h, RT
Urethral	1. Remove exudate from urethral orifice. 2. Collect discharge material on swab by massaging urethra against pubic symphysis through vagina.	Swab transport	≤2 h, RT	≤2 h, RT
Vaginal	1. Wipe away excessive amount of secretion or discharge. 2. Obtain secretions from mucosal membrane of vaginal vault with sterile swab.	Swab transport	≤2 h, RT	≤2 h, RT

	3. If smear is also requested, obtain it with second swab.		
Genital: female or male Lesion	1. Clean lesion with sterile saline, and remove lesion's surface with sterile scalpel blade. 2. Allow transudate to accumulate. 3. While pressing base of lesion, *firmly* sample exudate with sterile swab.	Swab transport	≤2 h, RT
Genital: male Prostate	1. Clean glans with soap and water. 2. Massage prostate through rectum. 3. Collect fluid on sterile swab or in sterile tube.	Swab transport or sterile tube	≤2 h, RT
Urethral	Insert urethrogenital swab ≈1 in. (≈2.5 cm) into urethral lumen, rotate swab, and leave it in place for at least 2 s.	Swab transport	≤2 h, RT

(continued)

Specimen Collection

Specimen Collection

Table 3.1 General specimen collection and transport guidelines for bacteria and fungi[a] *(continued)*

| Specimen type | Collection | | Time and temp | |
	Guidelines	Device and/or minimum vol	Transport	Storage
Hair: dermatophytosis	1. With forceps, collect at least 10–12 affected hairs with bases of shafts intact. 2. Place in clean tube or container.	Clean container, 10 hairs	≤24 h, RT	
Nail: dermatophytosis	1. Wipe nail with 70% alcohol. Use gauze (not cotton). 2. Clip away generous portion of affected area, and collect material or debris from under nail. 3. Place material in clean container.	Clean container, enough scrapings to cover head of thumbtack	≤24 h, RT	
Pilonidal cyst	See Abscess.			
Respiratory tract, lower BAL, BBW, tracheal aspirate	1. Place aspirate or washing into sputum trap. 2. Place brush in sterile container with saline.	Sterile container, >1 ml	≤2 h, RT	≤24 h, 4°C

Sputum, expectorate	1. Collect specimen under *direct* supervision of nurse or physician. 2. Have patient rinse or gargle with water. Discard. 3. Instruct patient to cough *deeply* to produce lower respiratory tract specimen (not postnasal fluid). Collect into sterile container.	Sterile container, >1 ml	≤2 h, RT	≤24 h, 4°C
Sputum, induced	1. Have patient rinse mouth with water after brushing gums and tongue. 2. With aid of nebulizer, have patient inhale ≈25 ml of 3–10% sterile saline. 3. Collect induced sputum into sterile container.	Sterile container	≤2 h, RT	≤24 h, 4°C
Respiratory tract, upper Oral	1. Remove oral secretions or debris from surface of lesion with swab, and discard swab. 2. Using second swab, vigorously sample lesion, avoiding any areas of healthy tissue.	Swab transport	≤2 h, RT	≤24 h, RT

(continued)

Specimen Collection

Specimen Collection

Table 3.1 General specimen collection and transport guidelines for bacteria and fungi[a] (continued)

Specimen type	Collection		Time and temp	
	Guidelines	Device and/or minimum vol	Transport	Storage
Nasal	1. Use swab premoistened with sterile saline. Insert ≈1 in. (≈2.5 cm) into nares. 2. Rotate swab against nasal mucosa.	Swab transport	≤2 h, RT	≤24 h, RT
Nasopharyngeal	1. Gently insert calcium alginate swab into posterior nasopharynx via nose. 2. Rotate swab slowly for 5 s to absorb secretions. Remove swab. Inoculate medium at bedside, or place swab in transport medium.	Direct medium inoculation or swab transport	Plates: ≤15 min, RT Swabs: ≤2 h, RT	≤24 h, RT
Throat	1. Depress tongue with tongue depressor. 2. Sample posterior pharynx, tonsils, and inflamed areas with sterile swab.	Swab transport	≤2 h, RT	≤24 h, RT
Skin: dermatophytosis	1. Cleanse affected area with 70% alcohol. 2. Gently scrape surface of skin at *active margin* of lesion. *Do not draw blood.*	Clean container, enough scrapings to cover head of thumbtack	≤24 h, RT	

Specimen	Collection procedure	Transport container		
Tissue	3. Place sample in clean container.			
	1. Submit in sterile container.	Anaerobic transport system	≤15 min, RT	≤24 h, RT
	2. For small samples, add several drops of sterile saline to keep moist.			
	3. *Do not allow tissue to dry out.*			
	4. Place in anaerobic transport system.			
Urine Female, midstream	1. Thoroughly clean urethral area with soap and water.	Sterile wide-mouth container, ≥1 ml, or urine transport kit	Unpreserved: ≤2 h, RT	≤24 h, 4°C; preserved, ≤24 h, RT
	2. Rinse area with wet gauze pads.			
	3. While holding labia apart, begin voiding.			
	4. After several ml has passed, collect midstream portion without stopping flow of urine.			
Male, midstream	1. Clean glans with soap and water.	Sterile wide-mouth container, ≥1 ml, or urine transport kit	Unpreserved: ≤2 h, RT	≤24 h, 4°C; preserved, ≤24 h, RT
	2. Rinse area with wet gauze pads.			
	3. While holding foreskin retracted, begin voiding.			
	4. After several ml has passed, collect midstream portion without stopping flow of urine.			

(continued)

Specimen Collection

Specimen Collection

Table 3.1 General specimen collection and transport guidelines for bacteria and fungi[a] *(continued)*

| Specimen type | Collection | | Time and temp | |
	Guidelines	Device and/or minimum vol	Transport	Storage
Straight catheter	1. Thoroughly clean urethral area with soap and water. 2. Rinse area with wet gauze pads. 3. Aseptically insert catheter into bladder. 4. Allow ≈15 ml to pass. Then collect urine to be submitted in sterile container.	Sterile leakproof container	Unpreserved: ≤2 h, RT	≤24 h, 4°C; preserved, ≤24 h, RT
Indwelling catheter	1. Disinfect catheter collection port with 70% alcohol. 2. Use needle and syringe to aseptically collect 5–10 ml of urine. 3. Transfer sample to sterile tube or container.	Sterile leakproof container	Unpreserved: ≤2 h, RT	≤24 h, 4°C; preserved, ≤24 h, RT
Foley catheter	See Catheter, Foley			
Wound	See Abscess.			

[a] Abbreviations: AFB, acid-fast bacilli; BAL, bronchoalveolar lavage; BBW, bronchial brushing or washing; i.v., intravenous; RT, room temperature.

Table 3.2 Selection of specimens and tests to confirm infectious food-borne diseases[a]

Disease	Specimens and tests
Bacterial	
Bacillus cereus gastroenteritis	Isolation of same serotype of *B. cereus* from stool specimens from most ill persons but not from controls
	Isolation of $\geq 10^5$ *B. cereus*/g of epidemiologically implicated food
	Detection of enterotoxin by ligated rabbit ileal loop, vascular permeability reaction, immunogel-diffusion, aggregate-hemagglutination, or reverse passive latex agglutination
	Detection of emetic enterotoxin by HEp-2 cell test
Botulism	Isolation of *Clostridium botulinum* from stool of ill person who ate epidemiologically implicated food
	Detection of botulinal toxin in sera, feces, or food by mouse test
	Typical clinical syndrome in persons known to have eaten same epidemiologically implicated foods as person with laboratory-proven cases
	Suspicion is cast when patients have typical clinical syndrome and history of eating home-canned or home-fermented fish, roe, or sea mammal meat.
Brucellosis	Isolation of *Brucella* spp. from blood of ill persons
	Fourfold or greater increase in agglutination titer between blood specimens taken during acute illness and 3 to 6 wk after onset of illness

(continued)

Specimen Collection

Table 3.2 Selection of specimens and tests to confirm infectious food-borne diseases[a] *(continued)*

Disease	Specimens and tests
Campylobacteriosis	Isolation of *Campylobacter jejuni* from stools of most ill persons or from epidemiologically implicated food
	Same strains in patients and food according to bacterial restriction endonuclease DNA analysis
	Fourfold or greater rise of agglutination titer between blood specimens taken during acute illness and 2 to 4 wk after onset of illness
Cholera	Isolation of *Vibrio cholerae* from vomitus or stool of ill person who ate epidemiologically implicated foods
	Isolation of *V. cholerae* from epidemiologically implicated food
	Rise of vibriocidal, antitoxin, or bacterial agglutinating antibody titer during acute or early convalescent phases of illness and fall of titer during convalescent phase in nonimmunized persons
	Demonstration of culture or filtrate to be enterotoxigenic by gut loop, infant mouse cell culture, or other biological technique
	Suspicion is cast when patients have typical clinical syndrome and history of eating raw seafoods.
Clostridium perfringens enteritis	Fecal spore count of >10^6/g in most ill persons examined within few days of illness onset
	Isolation of same serotype of *C. perfringens* from specimens from most ill persons but not from controls
	Isolation of same serotype of *C. perfringens* from ill persons and epidemiologically implicated food
	Isolation of ≥10^5 *C. perfringens*/g of epidemiologically implicated food

Escherichia coli diarrhea	Demonstration of toxin in feces by reverse passive hemagglutination and fluorescent-antibody techniques
	Isolation of same serotype of *E. coli* (known to be enterotoxigenic, enteroinvasive, enterohemolytic, or enteropathogenic) from stool specimens from most ill persons but not from controls
	Isolation of same serotype of *E. coli* (known to be enterotoxigenic, enteroinvasive, enterohemolytic, or enteropathogenic) from ill persons and from epidemiologically implicated food
	Demonstration of toxin to be:
	Enterotoxigenic by ileal loop (LT), infant mouse (ST), Y1 adrenal cell culture (LT), ELISA, or T and ST genes
	Invasive by production Sereny test, HeLa cell tissue culture, or genes for invasive proteins
	Enterohemorrhagic by infant rabbit model, Vero or endothelial cell, tissue culture, ELISA, other immunoassays, enterotoxin, or adhesion genes
	Enteroadherent by HEp-2 cell tissue assay or aggregative-adherence genes
	Enteropathogenic by HEp-2 cell tissue assay or focal adherence genes
Listeriosis	Isolation of *Listeria monocytogenes* from autopsy or fetal material of fatal case
	Isolation of same phage type (from same serogroup) of culture isolated from patients and food
	(Virulence of strains is tested by Anton test in rabbits, inoculation of mice, and inoculation of embryonated eggs.)
Salmonellosis	Isolation of *Salmonella* spp. from stool or rectal swab (urine or blood if septicemic symptoms occur) of ill persons
	Isolation of *Salmonella* spp. from epidemiologically implicated food
	Isolation of same *Salmonella* serovar from ill persons and from epidemiologically implicated food

(continued)

Specimen Collection

Table 3.2 Selection of specimens and tests to confirm infectious food-borne diseases[a] *(continued)*

Disease	Specimens and tests
Shigellosis	Isolation of *Shigella* serovars from stool or rectal swab of ill persons
	Isolation of *Shigella* serovars from epidemiologically implicated food
	Isolation of same *Shigella* serovar from ill persons and from epidemiologically implicated food (and from stool of food worker)
Staphylococcal enterotoxicosis (intoxication) or food poisoning	Detection of enterotoxin in epidemiologically implicated food by serological assay
	Isolation of same phage type of specimen from ill person and from epidemiologically implicated food (and skin, nose, or lesion of food worker)
	Isolation of $\geq 10^5$ *Staphylococcus aureus*/g of epidemiologically implicated food
Streptococcal sore throat or scarlet fever or diarrhea	Isolation of same M and T types of group A or G streptococci from throats of ill persons and epidemiologically implicated food
Vibrio cholerae non-O1 gastroenteritis	Isolation of *V. cholerae* of same serotype from stools of ill persons
	Isolation of *V. cholerae* from epidemiologically implicated food
Vibrio parahaemolyticus gastroenteritis	Isolation of Kanagawa-positive *V. parahaemolyticus* of same serotype from stool of most ill persons
	Isolation of $\geq 10^5$ *V. parahaemolyticus* from epidemiologically implicated food
Vibrio vulnificus septicemia	Isolation of *V. vulnificus* from blood of ill person

Yersiniosis	Isolation of *Yersinia enterocolitica* or *Yersinia pseudotuberculosis* from stool or blood of most ill persons
	Isolation of *Y. enterocolitica* or *Y. pseudotuberculosis* from epidemiologically implicated food
	Fourfold or greater rise of agglutination titer between blood specimens taken during acute illness and 2 to 4 wk after onset of illness
Viral	
Hepatitis A	Detection of IgM anti-hepatitis A virus from persons who ate epidemiologically implicated foods
	Observation of typical virus by immunoelectron microscopy (impractical in most laboratories)
	Titer rise (Fourfold rise is difficult to demonstrate unless patient is seen early in course of illness.)
	Suspicion is cast when adult patients have history of recent ingestion of raw shellfish.
Norwalk and parvo-like viral diseases	Serological evidence of virus
	Fourfold or greater rise of antibody titer of sera from acute phase to convalescent phase
	Observation of typical small, round, structured virus by immunoelectron microscopy confirmed by testing with reference antisera (impractical in most laboratories)
	Suspicion is cast when patients have syndrome, incubation period, and duration of illness compatible with typically described illness.

(continued)

Specimen Collection

Table 3.2 Selection of specimens and tests to confirm infectious food-borne diseases[a] *(continued)*

Disease	Specimens and tests
Parasitic	
Cryptosporidiosis	Isolation of *Cryptosporidium* spp. from most ill persons plus either food association or isolation from implicated food
	Large no. of oocysts in stools of ill persons
	Developmental stages in jejunal, ileal, or colonic biopsy
	Serum antibody
Giardiasis	Demonstration of *Giardia lamblia* in stool, duodenal contents, or small-bowel biopsy sample
	Detection of antigen in stool of patients
Trichinellosis	Recovery of trichinella cysts from deltoid or gastrocnemius muscle biopsy sample
	Demonstration of larva in epidemiologically implicated food
	Serological evidence of infection
	Suspicion is cast when patients have typical syndrome and history of eating pork, bear, or Arctic mammals.

Fungal

Amanitotoxin, phallin, or gyromitrin group mushroom poisoning	Demonstration of amanitotoxin, phallin, or gyromitrin in urine or in epidemiologically implicated mushrooms
	Suspicion is cast when patients have history of eating gathered mushrooms.
Gastroenteritis-causing group mushroom poisoning	Demonstration of toxic chemical in epidemiologically implicated mushrooms
	Suspicion is cast when patients have history of eating gathered mushrooms.
Ibotenic acid and muscimol group mushroom poisoning	Demonstration of ibotenic acid or muscimol in epidemiologically implicated mushrooms
	Suspicion is cast when patients have history of eating gathered mushrooms.
Mushroom-alcohol intolerance	Demonstration of toxic chemicals in urine or in epidemiologically implicated mushrooms
	Suspicion is cast when patients have history of eating gathered mushrooms and drinking alcohol within 24 h.
Muscarine group mushroom poisoning	Demonstration of muscarine in urine or in epidemiologically implicated mushrooms
	Suspicion is cast when patients have history of eating gathered mushrooms.

[a] Abbreviations: ELISA, enzyme-linked immunosorbent assay; IgM, immunoglobulin M; LT, heat-labile enterotoxin; ST, heat-stable enterotoxin; T, toxin.

Specimen Collection

Specimen Collection

Table 3.3 Preservatives[a]

Preservative	Advantages	Disadvantages
5 or 10% formalin (buffered or not buffered)	Good stool fixative for concentrates; easy to prepare; long shelf life. Concentrated sediments can be used with new monoclonal detection kits and for acid-fast stains.	Not good for direct wet mount; does not preserve trophozoites; does not preserve organism morphology for acceptable permanent stained smear. Formaldehyde vapors must be monitored.
Merthiolate-iodine-formalin	Components both fix and stain organisms for wet mounts. Easy to prepare; long shelf life; contains no mercury compounds; useful for field surveys	Not good for direct wet mount; organism morphology on permanent stained smears generally not as good as that seen with Schaudinn's fluid or PVA (mercuric chloride base). Formaldehyde vapors must be monitored.
Sodium acetate-acetic acid formalin	Used for concentration and permanent stained smears; contains no mercury compounds; easy to prepare; long shelf life. Concentrated sediment can be used with new monoclonal detection kits or for acid-fast stains.	Albumin-glycerin required for adhesion of specimen to slide; not good for direct wet mount; organism morphology on stained smears better with iron hematoxylin stains than with trichrome. Formaldehyde vapors must be monitored.

Fixative		
Schaudinn's fixative	Used for smears prepared from fresh specimens from intestinal mucosal surfaces; excellent preservation of protozoan trophozoites and cysts	Not recommended for use in wet mounts or procedures; contains mercuric chloride; poor adhesive qualities with liquid or mucoid specimens
PVA in Schaudinn's fixative	Excellent preservation of protozoan trophozoites and cysts for permanent stained smears, which can be prepared in ~1 h or 1 wk or some no later; good adhesion to slide; long shelf life. Specimen can be concentrated but not as well as formalin-preserved specimens.	Contains mercuric chloride (Schaudinn's fluid); difficult to prepare in laboratory; not as good as formalin for concentration procedures; cannot use specimens with monoclonal detection kits or acid-fast stains
Modified PVA (copper, zinc bases)	Can prepare permanent stained smears and perform concentration techniques; does not contain mercury compounds	Protozoan morphology poor when preserved in copper sulfate-based PVA; morphology better with zinc sulfate-based PVA. Organisms may be difficult to see, but with experience, they can be identified.

[a] PVA, polyvinyl alcohol.

Specimen Collection

*Specimen
Processing*

This section is subdivided into parts describing

- primary plating media for bacteria, mycobacteria, and fungi;
- dyes and pH indicators;
- tissue culture cell lines for virus and *Chlamydia* isolation;
- principles of staining procedures for bacteria, fungi, and parasites; and
- recommendations for processing specimens for bacteria, fungi, viruses, and parasites.

The recommendations for processing specimens are limited to general guidelines. Consult the *Manual of Clinical Microbiology, Clinical Microbiology Procedures Handbook,* or other reference text for recommendations on isolating specific pathogens.

Primary Plating Media: Bacteria

Bacteroides Bile Esculin (BBE) Agar

Bacteroides bile esculin agar is a selective, differential agar medium used for the recovery of the *Bacteroides fragilis* group. The medium contains oxgall (bile), esculin, ferric ammonium citrate, hemin, vitamin K_1, and gentamicin in a casein and soybean agar base. Growth of non-*B. fragilis* group organisms is inhibited by the bile and the gentamicin. Supplementation of the agar with hemin and vitamin K_1 stimulates the growth of *Bacteroides* spp. Esculin hydrolysis is detected when esculin is converted to esculetin and reacts with ferric ammonium citrate to produce black colonies.

Bile-Esculin (Enterococcal Selective) Agar

Bile-esculin agar can be made selective for the recovery of vancomycin-resistant enterococci by adding vancomycin (e.g., 6 μg/ml) to it. Enterococci are able to grow and hydrolyze esculin in the presence of bile. Vancomycin-resistant strains produce black colonies on this agar, but susceptible strains fail to grow.

Blood Agar

Many types of blood agar media are used in clinical laboratories. The two basic components are the basal medium (e.g., brain heart infusion, brucella, Columbia, Schaedler's, tryptic soy) and blood (e.g., sheep, horse, rabbit). Additional supplements are commonly used to enhance the growth of specific organisms or to suppress the growth of unwanted organisms.

Bordet-Gengou (BG) Agar

Recovery of *Bordetella pertussis* and *Bordetella parapertussis* is inhibited by factors such as fatty acids, metal ions, sulfides, and peroxides that are commonly present in media. Starch, charcoal, serum albumin, blood, or similar components must be added to the medium to neutralize these inhibitors. Bordet-Gengou agar is a potato-infusion-glycerol-based agar medium supplemented with 20 to 30% sheep blood. Potato infusion is required for the growth of *Bordetella* spp., and glycerol is added to conserve moisture in the medium. Antibiotics such as methicillin and cephalexin are commonly added to suppress the growth of bacteria such as staphylococci, which inhibit the growth of *Bordetella* spp. Because this medium must be made fresh (shelf life of less than 1 week), it has largely been replaced by Regan-Lowe agar.

Buffered Charcoal-Yeast Extract (BCYE) Agar

Buffered charcoal-yeast extract agar is selective for the recovery of *Legionella* and *Nocardia* spp. It contains agar, yeast extract, charcoal, and salts and is supplemented with L-cysteine, ferric pyrophosphate, ACES [*N*-(2-acetamido)-2-aminoethanesulfonic acid] buffer, and α-ketoglutarate. The charcoal detoxifies the medium, the yeast extracts are rich in nutrients, and L-cysteine, ferric pyrophosphate, and α-ketoglutarate stimulate the growth of *Legionella* spp. The addition of ACES is required to buffer the medium, because *Legionella* spp. have a narrow pH tolerance (growth is optimal at pH 6.9). Antibiotics such as polymyxin B, anisomycin, and either cefamandole or vancomycin are added to inhibit the growth of other bacteria when nonsterile specimens are cultured.

Campylobacter Selective Medium

A large number of media have been developed for the selective isolation of campylobacters from stool specimens. Most of these media use a brucella basal medium, which preferentially supports the growth of *Campylobacter* spp. Blood is added, as are various combinations of antibiotics (e.g., cephalothin, vancomycin, trimethoprim, amphotericin, and polymyxin in the Blaser-Wang formulation; cycloheximide, cefazolin, novobiocin, bacitracin, and colistin in the Butzler formulation; cycloheximide, cefoperazone, and vancomycin in the Karmali formulation; cycloheximide, rifampin, trimethoprim, and polymyxin in the Preston formulation).

Cefsulodin-Irgasan-Novobiocin (CIN) Agar

Cefsulodin-Irgasan-novobiocin agar is a selective, differential agar medium used for the isolation of *Yersinia* and *Aeromonas* spp. The medium consists of digests of animal tissue and gelatin, beef and yeast extracts, sodium pyruvate, sodium deoxycholate, neutral red, crystal violet, cefsulodin, Irgasan, and novobiocin. The antibiotics and sodium deoxycholate inhibit the growth of most organisms in stool specimens. However, *Yersinia enterocolitica* and *Aeromonas* spp. are resistant and are able to ferment mannitol in the medium. This fermentation produces colonies with a bull's eye appearance, i.e., deep red centers with transparent edges.

Chocolate Agar

Chocolate agar is an enriched medium that derives its name from its color. Blood or hemoglobin is added immediately after the medium is heated, and the heat causes the added component to lyse and turn brown. This medium supports the growth of most bacteria and is required for the recovery of many species of *Haemophilus* and some pathogenic strains of *Neisseria*. A variety of formulations of this medium have been used, but the most common consists of a peptone base enriched with 2% hemoglobin or IsoVitaleX. Catalase-negative bacteria (e.g., *Streptococcus pneumoniae*) grow less well on this medium than on blood agar, because catalase from erythrocytes in the blood agar is not available to protect the bacteria from peroxides that accumulate in the medium.

Chopped Meat Broth

Chopped meat broth is an enriched broth used for the recovery of a variety of bacteria, particularly anaerobes, from clinical specimens. Extracts as well as solid particles of beef or horse meat are suspended in broth with peptones, yeast extract, sugars, starch, and L-cysteine. The L-cysteine helps maintain a low E_h (oxidation-reduction potential), which supports the growth of anaerobes.

Colistin-Nalidixic Acid (CNA) Agar

Colistin-nalidixic acid selective medium is used for the recovery of aerobic and anaerobic gram-positive bacteria. The medium consists of Columbia agar base supplemented with nalidixic acid, colistin, and blood. Nalidixic acid inhibits most aerobic gram-negative bacilli, as does colistin. The *B. fragilis* group is usually resistant to these antibiotics, but other anaerobic gram-negative bacilli can be inhibited by colistin.

Cycloserine-Cefoxitin-Egg Yolk-Fructose Agar (CCFA)

Cycloserine-cefoxitin-egg yolk-fructose agar is a selective, differential agar medium used for the recovery of *Clostridium difficile*. The medium consists of animal tissue digest, fructose, cycloserine, cefoxitin, and neutral red. Cycloserine and cefoxitin inhibit most intestinal bacteria. *C. difficile* can ferment fructose, producing an acid shift in pH that is detected by the indicator dye neutral red (the medium surrounding the colonies changes from red to yellow). Various modifications of this medium, including supplementation with egg yolk to stimulate growth of clostridia, are used.

Eosin-Methylene Blue (EMB) Agar

Eosin-methylene blue agar is a differential, selective medium used for the isolation and differentiation of lactose- and non-lactose-fermenting gram-negative bacilli. The agar medium consists of casein digests, lactose, sucrose, eosin Y, and methylene blue. The Levine formulation does not include sucrose. The growth of gram-positive bacteria is suppressed by methylene blue, which together with eosin Y also serves as an indicator of carbohydrate fermentation (dyes precipitate in an acid pH). The colonies of bacteria that ferment lactose (e.g., *Escherichia, Klebsiella,* and *Enterobacter* spp.) have a green metallic sheen or are blue-black to brown. Nonfermentative colonies (e.g., *Proteus, Salmonella,* and *Shigella* spp.) are colorless or light purple.

Fletcher Medium

Fletcher medium is a semisolid medium used for the recovery of *Leptospira* spp. The medium consists of 0.15% agar, salt, peptones, beef extract, and rabbit serum. Leptospires usually grow within 1 to 2 weeks in this medium.

Gram-Negative (Hajna; GN) Broth

Gram-negative broth is a selective enrichment broth for the recovery of small numbers of salmonellae and shigellae from stool specimens. The medium consists of digests of casein and animal tissues, mannitol, glucose, sodium citrate, and sodium deoxycholate. Sodium citrate and sodium deoxycholate inhibit the growth of many gram-positive and gram-negative bacteria.

The fact that the concentration of mannitol is higher than that of glucose limits the growth of *Proteus* spp. However, commensal organisms will overgrow the enteric pathogens if the broth is incubated for more than 4 to 6 h.

Hektoen Enteric (HE) Agar

Hektoen enteric agar is a selective medium used for the isolation of *Salmonella* and *Shigella* spp. and the differentiation of these organisms from other gram-negative bacilli that may be recovered on this medium. It consists of a peptone base agar supplemented with bile salts, lactose, sucrose, salicin, ferric ammonium citrate, and the pH indicators bromthymol blue and acid fuchsin. The bile inhibits all gram-positive bacteria and many gram-negative bacilli. Acids produced by fermentation of lactose, sucrose, or salicin react with bromthymol blue to produce a yellow color and with acid fuchsin to produce a red color. Hydrogen sulfide produced by the metabolism of sodium thiosulfate is detected when a black precipitate is produced by the addition of ferric ammonium citrate. Lactose-fermenting bacteria (e.g., *Escherichia coli*) are slightly inhibited on this agar and appear as orange or salmon pink colonies. *Salmonella* colonies are typically blue-green with black center. *Shigella* colonies are green with no black centers. *Proteus* spp. are inhibited; their colonies are colorless.

Kanamycin-Vancomycin Laked (LKV) Blood Agar

Kanamycin-vancomycin laked blood agar is a selective, differential agar medium used for the recovery of anaerobic gram-negative bacilli, especially *Bacteroides* and *Prevotella* spp. The medium consists of casein and soybean meal agar supplemented with kanamycin, vancomycin, vitamin K_1, and lysed (laked) sheep blood. Kanamycin inhibits most facultative gram-negative bacilli, and vancomycin inhibits most gram-positive organisms and *Porphyromonas* spp. Vitamin K_1 stimulates the growth of some *Prevotella* strains, which also develop a black pigment in the presence of lysed blood.

Kelly Medium

Kelly medium is used for the isolation of *Borrelia* species from human specimens and arthropod vectors. The success of these cultures depends on the quality of the medium. In general, specimens should be submitted to reference laboratories for processing. A modified version (i.e., Barbour-Stoenner-Kelly II medium) of the original formulation is currently used. The medium consists of peptone and casein digests, albumin, gelatin, rabbit serum, hemin, yeast extracts, glucose, and a complex mixture of buffers, amino acids, vitamins, nucleotides, and other growth factors. Kanamycin and 5-fluorouracil have been added to the medium for the selective isolation of borreliae from contaminated specimens. Recovery of the organisms requires prolonged incubation in a microaerophilic atmosphere at 30 to 37°C. Organisms are detected by examining the broth at weekly intervals by dark-field microscopy.

MacConkey (MAC) Agar

MacConkey agar is a selective agar medium used for the isolation and differentiation of lactose- and non-lactose-fermenting gram-negative bacilli. The medium consists of digests of peptones, bile salts, lactose, neutral red, and crystal violet. Bile salts and crystal violet inhibit the growth of gram-positive bacteria and some fastidious gram-negative bacteria. Colonies that ferment lactose (e.g., *Escherichia, Klebsiella,* and *Enterobacter* spp.) produce acids that cause a red color shift in the neutral red pH indicator and precipitate the bile salts. These colonies appear red to pink, while nonfermenting colonies (e.g., *Proteus, Salmonella,* and *Shigella* spp.) appear yellow, colorless, or translucent.

Mannitol Salt Agar

Mannitol salt agar is a selective agar medium used for the isolation of staphylococci. The medium consists of digests of casein and animal tissue, beef extract, mannitol, salt, and phenol red indicator. If the organism can grow in the presence of 7.5% salt and ferment mannitol, then the acid turns the indicator yellow. Most strains of *Staphylococcus aureus* produce yellow colonies, but coagulase-negative species of staphylococci do not ferment the mannitol and thus remain red. Most other organisms are inhibited by the high salt concentration.

New York City (NYC) Agar

New York City agar is a selective agar medium used for the isolation of pathogenic *Neisseria* spp. The medium consists of peptones, cornstarch, yeast dialysate, glucose, hemoglobin, horse plasma, and a mixture of antibiotics (vancomycin, colistin, amphotericin B, and trimethoprim). This medium can be exchanged with Thayer-Martin agar.

Phenylethyl Alcohol (PEA) Blood Agar

Phenylethyl alcohol blood agar is a selective blood agar medium that consists of casein and soybean agar supplemented with

Specimen Processing

phenylethyl alcohol and blood. Facultative gram-negative bacilli are inhibited by phenylethyl alcohol (e.g., the growth of
swarming *Proteus* spp is suppressed). Most gram-positive and
gram-negative anaerobes, as well as aerobic gram-positive bacteria, will grow on this medium. *Pseudomonas* spp are not inhibited on this medium.

Pseudomonas cepacia (PC) Agar

PC agar is a selective, differential medium used for the isolation
of *Burkholderia (Pseudomonas) cepacia* from clinical specimens contaminated with other organisms. The medium consists
of salt solutions, phosphate buffer, pyruvate, proteose peptones,
bile, crystal violet, ticarcillin, polymyxin B, and phenol red.
Burkholderia spp. are able to grow on this medium and metabol-
ize pyruvate, producing alkaline by-products. Hot pink to red
colonies are observed after 2 days of incubation. Other bacteria
are inhibited by the crystal violet and antibiotics.

Regan-Lowe (RL) Medium

Regan-Lowe agar medium, for the selective isolation of *Bordetella* spp., contains beef extract, gelatin digest, starch, charcoal,
niacin, 10% horse blood, and cephalexin (40 μg/ml). The charcoal and horse blood are required to neutralize fatty acids and
other inhibitory factors in the medium. Sheep but not human
blood can replace horse blood. Cephalexin can delay the detection of *Bordetella* spp. on this medium, but the use of an additional nonselective medium is not considered necessary. The
shelf life of this medium is 6 to 8 weeks.

Salmonella-Shigella (SS) Agar

Salmonella-shigella is a highly selective agar medium for the
recovery of *Salmonella* and *Shigella* spp. The medium consists
of beef extract and peptone digests, lactose as a carbohydrate
source, bile salts, sodium citrate, sodium thiosulfate, neutral
red, brilliant green, and ferric citrate. Bile salts, sodium citrate,
and brilliant green are inhibitory for all gram-positive and selected gram-negative bacteria. Bacteria that grow on the medium and produce hydrogen sulfide from the metabolism of
sodium thiosulfate are detected by the black precipitate formed
with ferric citrate. Acid produced by lactose fermentation is
detected with the pH indicator neutral red. All lactose-fermenting colonies appear pink or red, and non-lactose-fermenting
colonies appear either colorless (e.g., *Shigella* spp.) or black
(e.g., *Salmonella* spp.).

Selenite Broth

Selenite broth is a selective enrichment broth used for the isolation of *Salmonella* spp. from stools and other contaminated specimens. The medium consists of peptones, sodium phosphate, lactose, and sodium selenite. *E. coli* and other gram-negative bacilli are inhibited by sodium selenite. The broth should be subcultured within 8 to 12 h after inoculation with the specimen, or else the enteric pathogens will be overgrown with commensal organisms.

Sorbitol-MacConkey Agar

Sorbitol-MacConkey agar is a selective differential agar used for the isolation of *E. coli* O157. Lactose is replaced with sorbitol. Most *E. coli* strains ferment sorbitol; however, *E. coli* O157 does not ferment sorbitol, and therefore its colonies are colorless on this agar.

Tetrathionate Broth

Tetrathionate broth is a selective enrichment broth used for the recovery of *Salmonella* spp. from stool specimens. It consists of a peptone base supplemented with yeast extract, mannitol, glucose, sodium deoxycholate, sodium thiosulfate, calcium carbonate, and brilliant green. Sodium deoxycholate, sodium thiosulfate, and brilliant green inhibit gram-positive and gram-negative bacteria. The broth should be subcultured 12 to 24 h after inoculation to prevent overgrowth of *Salmonella* spp. with commensal organisms.

Thayer-Martin (Modified) (MTM) Agar

Many modifications of Thayer-Martin medium have been developed for the isolation of pathogenic neisseriae. The blood agar base medium is enriched with hemoglobin and supplements. The growth of unwanted bacteria can be suppressed by the addition of antibiotics such as colistin (inhibits most gram-negative bacteria except *Proteus* spp.), trimethoprim (inhibits *Proteus* spp.), vancomycin (inhibits most gram-positive bacteria), and nystatin (inhibits yeasts). Some strains of *Neisseria gonorrhoeae* are inhibited by vancomycin, so nonselective media (e.g. chocolate agar) should also be used for isolation.

Thioglycolate Broth

Thioglycolate broth is an enrichment broth used for the recovery of aerobic and anaerobic bacteria. Various formulations are used, but most include casein digest, glucose, yeast extract, cysteine, and sodium thioglycolate. Supplementation with hemin and vitamin K_1 enhances the recovery of anaerobic bacteria.

Thiosulfate Citrate Bile Salt Sucrose (TCBS) Agar

Thiosulfate citrate bile salt sucrose agar is a selective, differential agar medium used for the recovery of *Vibrio* spp. The medium consists of digests of casein and animal tissue, yeast extract, sodium citrate, sodium cholate, oxgall (bile), sucrose, ferric citrate, thymol blue, and bromthymol blue. Sodium citrate, sodium cholate, and bile inhibit commensal organisms. *Vibrio cholerae* colonies are yellow on this medium because fermentation of sucrose by the acid results in a yellow color shift of the indicator bromthymol blue. *Vibrio parahaemolyticus* fails to ferment sucrose, and its colonies are therefore blue-green. Some enteric bacilli and enterococci may grow, but their colonies are usually small and translucent. Sucrose-fermenting *Proteus* strains produce yellow colonies that are similar to *Vibrio* colonies.

Tinsdale Agar

Tinsdale agar is a selective differential medium used for the isolation of *Corynebacterium diphtheriae* from upper respiratory tract specimens. The medium consists of peptones, salt, yeast extract, L-cysteine, potassium tellurite, and serum. Potassium tellurite inhibits the growth of most commensal organisms in the upper respiratory tract and allows the growth of *C. diphtheriae* and related *Corynebacterium* species. *C. diphtheriae* colonies can be distinguished by the brown halos that develop around the black colonies. These halos result from the reaction of tellurite with hydrogen sulfide, which *C. diphtheriae* produces from the cysteine in the medium.

Xylose-Lysine-Deoxycholate (XLD) Agar

Xylose-lysine-deoxycholate agar is a moderately selective agar medium used for the isolation and differentiation of enteric pathogens. The medium consists of yeast extract with xylose, lysine, lactose, sucrose, sodium deoxycholate, sodium thiosulfate, ferric ammonium citrate, and phenol red. The majority of the nonpathogenic enteric bacilli ferment lactose, sucrose, or xylose and produce yellow colonies (phenol red indicator is yellow at an acidic pH). Because *Shigella* spp. do not ferment these carbohydrates, their colonies are red. *Salmonella* and *Edwardsiella* spp. ferment xylose, but they also decarboxylate lysine to an alkaline diamine, cadaverine. This diamine neutralizes the acid products of fermentation and produces red colonies. If the organism produces hydrogen sulfide (e.g., *Salmonella* and *Edwardsiella* spp.), the centers of the colonies will blacken. Sodium deoxycholate inhibits the growth of many nonpathogenic organisms (in the presence of acid, sodium deoxycholate precipitates and produces yellow, opaque colonies).

Primary Plating Media: Mycobacteria

American Thoracic Society Medium

American Thoracic Society medium contains coagulated egg yolks, potato flour, glycerol, and malachite green. The concentration of malachite green is lower than that in Lowenstein-Jensen (LJ) medium, thus allowing earlier detection of mycobacterial colonies, but the medium is also more easily overgrown by contaminants.

BACTEC 12B Broth

BACTEC 12B broth is used in the BACTEC AFB automated culture system. The formulation is Middlebrook 7H9 broth supplemented with albumin, casein hydrolysate, catalase, and ^{14}C-labeled palmitic acid. As the mycobacteria grow, palmitic acid is metabolized, and $^{14}CO_2$ is released and detected by the BACTEC instrument. Contaminating bacteria are suppressed by the addition of polymyxin B, nalidixic acid, trimethoprim, azlocillin, and polyoxylene stearate.

BACTEC 13A Broth

BACTEC 13A broth is also used in the BACTEC system. The formulation is Middlebrook 7H12 medium supplemented with sodium polyanetholesulfonate. This broth can be used for blood and bone marrow aspirate specimens.

Dubos Broth

Dubos broth, a nonselective broth, contains casein digests, salt solutions, L-asparagine, ferric ammonium citrate, albumin or serum, and Tween 80. The growth of most species of mycobacteria is rapid in this medium, although the addition of antibiotics is required when specimens from contaminated sites are processed. Tween 80 is a surfactant that facilitates the dispersal of clumps of mycobacteria and results in more rapid, homogeneous growth.

Lowenstein-Jensen (LJ) Medium

LJ medium consists of glycerol, potato flour, defined salts, and coagulated whole eggs (to solidify the medium). Malachite green is added to inhibit contaminating bacteria, particularly gram-positive bacteria. LJ medium has a long shelf life (several months) and supports the growth of most mycobacteria, in part because lecithin in the eggs neutralizes many toxic factors present in clinical specimens. A problem with this medium is that the contaminants that grow on LJ can completely hydrolyze the medium.

LJ Medium, Gruft Modification

The Gruft modification of LJ medium contains RNA, penicillin, and nalidixic acid, which further suppress the growth of contaminating organisms. Because the growth of mycobacteria can be delayed with this selective medium, it should always be used with a tube of nonselective medium.

LJ Medium, Mycobactosel Modification

The Mycobactosel modification of LJ medium contains cycloheximide, lincomycin, and nalidixic acid.

Middlebrook 7H9 Broth

The 7H9 formulation of Middlebrook broth medium is the same as Middlebrook 7H10 agar except that the agar and malachite green have been removed. The growth of most mycobacteria is rapid in this medium, although antibiotics must be added to suppress the growth of contaminants.

Middlebrook 7H10 Agar

Middlebrook 7H10 agar, a nonselective agar medium, contains defined salts, vitamins, cofactors, oleic acid, albumin, catalase, glycerol, glucose, and malachite green. The addition of glycerol enhances the growth of *Mycobacterium avium-intracellulare.* Pyruvic acid can be added if *Mycobacterium bovis* is suspected, and 0.25% L-asparagine or 0.1% potassium aspartate must be added for maximal production of niacin. The medium has a relatively short shelf life (approximately 1 month), and exposure to heat or light may result in deterioration of the medium and release of formaldehyde. Growth of mycobacteria can be detected earlier on this medium than on egg-based media.

Middlebrook 7H10 Agar, Mycobactosel Modification

The Mycobactosel modification of Middlebrook 7H10 medium contains malachite green, cycloheximide, lincomycin, and nalidixic acid. As with the selective LJ media, the presence of antibiotics may delay the detection of mycobacteria, so a nonselective isolation medium should also be used.

Middlebrook 7H11 Agar

Middlebrook 7H11 agar is preferred over 7H10 because the addition of casein hydrolysates improves the recovery of isoniazid-resistant strains of *Mycobacterium tuberculosis,* which have become prevalent in some communities.

Middlebrook 7H11 Agar, Mitchison's Modification

Mitchison's modification of 7H11 medium contains carbenicillin, polymyxin B, trimethoprim, and amphotericin B. The carbenicillin is particularly useful for suppressing the growth of *Pseudomonas* spp.

Middlebrook 7H13 Broth

Middlebrook 7H13 broth is based on the 7H9 broth formulation supplemented with casein hydrolysate, polysorbate 80, sodium polyanetholesulfonate, catalase, and [^{14}C]palmitic acid. This broth is used in the BACTEC system.

Petragnani Medium

Petragnani medium is a nonselective mycobacterial medium that contains coagulated whole eggs, egg yolks, whole milk, potato, potato flour, glycerol, and malachite green. This medium is more inhibitory than LJ medium because it contains a higher concentration of malachite green. It should be restricted to use with heavily contaminated specimens.

Primary Plating Media: Fungi

Brain Heart Infusion (BHI) Agar

Brain heart infusion agar is a nutritionally enriched agar medium that can be used to isolate a variety of fastidious bacteria, yeasts, and molds. It is prepared with infusions of calf brains and beef hearts, peptones, glucose, sodium chloride, and disodium phosphate. Supplementation with 5 to 10% sheep blood can enrich the medium, and the addition of antibiotics (e.g., gentamicin, chloramphenicol, penicillin) can made this medium selective for fungi.

Dermatophyte Test Medium (DTM)

Dermatophyte test medium is a selective agar medium used for the isolation and identification of dermatophytes. It consists of

digests of soybean meal supplemented with glucose, cycloheximide, chlortetracycline, gentamicin, and phenol red. The antibiotics suppress the growth of bacteria, saprophytic yeasts, and
molds. Dermatophytes growing on this medium produce alkaline by-products that change the phenol red indicator from yellow to red. This color change may be obscured when grossly
contaminated specimens (e.g., nails) are processed on this medium. The pigment produced by dermatophytes, which is used
for identifying them, is obscured by the intense red color produced on this medium.

Inhibitory Mold Agar (IMA)

Inhibitory mold agar is an enriched, selective agar medium used
for the isolation of pathogenic fungi other than dermatophytes.
It consists of digests of animal tissue and casein, yeast extract,
dextrin, starch, glucose, salts, and chloramphenicol. Contaminating bacteria are inhibited by chloramphenicol.

Mycosel (Mycobiotic) Agar

Mycosel (Mycobiotic) agar is a selective agar medium used for
the isolation of pathogenic fungi from contaminated specimens.
Mycosel agar (BBL) and Mycobiotic agar (Difco) consist of
digests of soybean meal supplemented with glucose, cycloheximide, and chloramphenicol. Cycloheximide-susceptible fungi,
including *Cryptococcus neoformans, Pseudallescheria boydii,*
the zygomycetes, many species of *Candida* and *Aspergillus,*
and most saprophytic or opportunistic fungi, will not grow on
this medium.

SABHI Blood Agar

Sabouraud agar-brain heart infusion (SABHI), an enriched agar
medium, is a variation of Sabouraud dextrose agar (described
below). The medium consists of infusions of beef hearts and
calf brains, peptones, salts, glucose, blood, and chloromycetin
(chloramphenicol). It is used for the cultivation of dermatophytes and other pathogenic and nonpathogenic fungi.

Sabouraud Dextrose Agar (SDA)

SDA is an enriched agar medium used for the isolation of saprophytic and pathogenic fungi. The original formulation of SDA
consists of digests of casein and animal tissue supplemented
with 4% glucose and adjusted to pH 5.6. The Emmons modification is preferred by many mycologists. It contains a reduced
concentration of glucose (2%) and is buffered to neutrality (pH
6.9). Yeasts, dermatophytes, and other filamentous fungi will

grow on these media. The original formulation of SDA was acidic to suppress the growth of bacteria. This acidity can be circumvented by the addition of antibiotics (e.g., cycloheximide, chloramphenicol) to the medium. However, cycloheximide-susceptible fungi (refer to Mycosel agar above) do not grow on this medium.

Yeast Extract-Phosphate Agar

Yeast extract-phosphate agar is a selective agar medium used for the isolation of pathogenic fungi such as *Histoplasma* and *Blastomyces* spp. It consists of yeast extract and phosphate buffer supplemented with chloramphenicol to suppress the growth of bacteria. The pH is adjusted to 6.0

Table 4.1 Dyes and pH indicators

Indicator	pH and color	
	Acid	Alkaline
Acid fuchsin (Andrade's)	5.0, pink	8.0, pale yellow
Bromcresol green	3.8, yellow	5.4, blue
Bromcresol purple	5.2, yellow	6.8, purple
Bromphenol blue	3.0, yellow	4.6, blue
Bromthymol blue	6.0, yellow	7.6, dark blue
Chlorcresol green	4.0, yellow	5.6, blue
Chlorphenol red	5.0, yellow	6.6, red
Cresolphthalein	8.2, colorless	9.8, red
m-Cresol purple	7.4, yellow	9.0, purple
Cresol red	7.2, yellow	8.8, red
Methyl red	4.4, red	6.2, yellow
Neutral red	6.8, red	8.0, yellow
Phenolphthalein	8.3, colorless	10.0, red
Phenol red	6.8, yellow	8.4, red
Thymol blue	8.0, yellow	9.6, blue
Resazurin	Oxidized: blue, nonfluorescent	Reduced: red, fluorescent
Triphenyl-tetrazolium chloride	Oxidized: colorless	Reduced: red

Specimen Processing

Specimen Processing

Table 4.2 Cells used for virus or *Chlamydia* isolation

Type of cell[a]	Species or tissue of origin	Virus(es) or *Chlamydia* sp. isolated
Primary cells		
African green monkey	Kidney	Herpes simplex viruses, mumps virus, respiratory syncytial virus, rubella virus, varicella-zoster virus
CBMC, PBMC	Human	Human immunodeficiency virus types 1 and 2, human T lymphotropic viruses 1 and 2, human herpesvirus 6
Chicken embryo fibroblasts	Chicken	Newcastle disease virus, human poxviruses
Embryonic kidney, lung	Human	Adenoviruses, human polyomavirus BK, mumps virus
Rabbit	Kidney	Herpes simplex virus
Rhesus or cynomolgus monkey	Kidney	Enteric cytopathic human orphan viruses, polioviruses, coxsackievirus groups A and B, mumps virus, reoviruses, influenza virus, measles virus, parainfluenza virus, respiratory syncytial virus
Finite cell lines		
Foreskin fibroblasts	Human	Cytomegalovirus, herpes simplex viruses
Kidney fibroblasts	Human, fetal	Coronaviruses, herpes simplex viruses, rhinoviruses
Lung fibroblasts	Human, embryo	Coronaviruses, cytomegalovirus, rhinoviruses, varicella-zoster virus
WI-38, MRC-5	Human fetal lung	Adenoviruses, cytomegalovirus, polioviruses, coxsackievirus group B, enteroviruses (types 68–71), respiratory syncytial virus, rhinoviruses

Continuous cell lines

293	Human kidney	Adenoviruses (types 5, 40, and 41)
A549	Human lung	Adenoviruses (types 1–39)
BGMK	Buffalo green monkey kidney	Poliovirus, coxsackievirus groups A and B, reoviruses, *C. trachomatis*
HeLa	Human cervix	*C. trachomatis, C. pneumoniae,* polioviruses, poxviruses, reoviruses, respiratory syncytial virus, rhinoviruses, coxsackievirus groups A and B
HEp-2	Human larynx	Adenoviruses, respiratory syncytial virus, *C. pneumoniae*
McCoy	Mouse	*C. trachomatis, C. psittaci*
MDCK	Canine kidney	Influenza virus, parainfluenza virus
Mink lung	Mink	Herpes simplex viruses
RD	Human rhabdomyosarcoma	Coronaviruses, coxsackievirus group A, polioviruses, enteroviruses (types 68–71)
RK$_{13}$	Rabbit kidney	Rubella virus, poxviruses
Vero, CV-1	African green monkey kidney	Herpes simplex viruses, measles virus, poxviruses, human polyomavirus BK, rubella virus, respiratory syncytial virus, parainfluenza virus

[a] CBMC, cord blood mononuclear cells; PBMC, peripheral blood mononuclear cells.

Specimen Processing

Microscopy

Specimen Processing

Acridine Orange Stain

Acridine orange is a fluorescent stain used for the detection of bacteria and fungi in clinical specimens. The dye intercalates into nucleic acid (native and denatured). At neutral pH, bacteria, fungi, and cellular material (e.g., leukocytes, squamous epithelial cells) stain red-orange. At acid pH (pH 4.0), bacteria and fungi remain red-orange but background material stains green-yellow.

Auramine-Rhodamine Stain

Auramine and rhodamine are fluorochromes that bind to mycolic acids and are resistant to decolorization with acid-alcohol (acid-fast stain). Acid-fast organisms appear orange-yellow. Potassium permanganate is used as a counterstain. It is a strong oxidizing agent that inactivates the unbound fluorochrome dyes to produce a black background for the stained specimens. Fluorochrome-stained smears can be restained by the Kinyoun or Ziehl-Neelsen methods.

Calcofluor White Stain

Calcofluor white is a nonspecific fluorochrome that binds to cellulose and chitin in the cell walls of fungi. The dye can be mixed with 10% potassium hydroxide so that mammalian cells can be dissolved, thus facilitating visualization of fungal elements. Fungi, *Pneumocystis* spp., and *Acanthamoeba* spp. appear green or blue against a dark background when the stained slide is examined under UV illumination. Care must be used to distinguish specific staining from stained debris.

Direct Fluorescent-Antibody Stain

A variety of organisms (e.g., *Streptococcus pyogenes*, *Bordetella pertussis*, *Francisella tularensis*, *Legionella* spp., *Chlamydia trachomatis*, *Cryptosporidium parvum*, *Giardia lamblia*, influenza virus, herpes simplex virus) are directly detected in clinical specimens by using specific fluorescein-labeled antibodies. The labeled antibodies bind to the organisms and fluoresce green under UV light. The sensitivity and specificity of the stain are determined by the quality of the antibodies used in the reagents.

Giemsa Stain

Giemsa stain, like Wright stain, is a modification of the Romanowsky stain, which combines methylene blue and eosin. Both stains are used for detection of blood parasites (e.g., *Plasmo-*

dium, Babesia, and *Leishmania* spp.), fungi (e.g., *Histoplasma* spp., yeast cells, *Pneumocystis* spp.), rickettsiae, chlamydiae, and viral inclusions. A protozoan trophozoite has a red nucleus and a gray-blue cytoplasm; intracellular yeasts and inclusions typically stain blue (basophilic); and rickettsiae, chlamydial elementary bodies, and *Pneumocystis* spp. stain purple.

Gram Stain

Gram stain is the most commonly used stain in clinical microbiology laboratories. It is used to separate bacteria into gram-positive (blue) and gram-negative (red) groups as well as to detect fungi and many parasites. Variations in the performance of this stain are commonplace, but the staining principle is constant. After fixation of the specimen to a glass slide (by heating or treatment with 95% methanol), the specimen is exposed to the basic dye, crystal violet. Iodine is added, and the iodine forms a complex with the primary dye. During the decolorization step, this complex is retained in gram-positive organisms but lost in gram-negative organisms. The gram-negative organisms are detected with a counterstain (e.g., safranin). The degree to which an organism retains the stain is a function of the species, culture conditions, and staining skills of the microbiologist. Older cultures tend to decolorize readily.

India Ink Stain (Nigrosin)

The use of India ink is not technically a staining method. Detection of an encapsulated fungus (e.g., *Cryptococcus neoformans*) is made possible by exclusion of the ink particles by the polysaccharide capsule of the organism. Care in interpretation is required because artifacts (e.g., leukocytes, erythrocytes, powder, bubbles) may be confused with yeast cells. The morphologic characteristics of the yeast cells must be recognized before the preparation can be interpreted.

Iron Hematoxylin Stain

Iron hematoxylin stain is used for the detection and identification of fecal protozoa. Helminth eggs and larvae generally retain too much stain and are more easily identified with wet-mount preparations. Iron hematoxylin stain can be applied to either fresh stool specimens or ones preserved with polyvinyl alcohol or a similar preservative. Formalin-fixed specimens cannot be used.

Kinyoun Stain

The presence of long-chain fatty acids (e.g., mycolic acid) in some organisms makes these organisms both difficult to stain with water-soluble dyes and resistant to decolorization with acid solutions (i.e., the organisms are considered acid-fast). The Kinyoun method of staining uses high concentrations of basic carbol fuchsin and phenol to facilitate penetration of the dye into the cells. This stain is also referred to as a cold acid-fast stain because the specimen does not need to be heated for the stain to penetrate, as it does with the Ziehl-Neelsen stain. Basic carbol fuchsin is used as the primary stain, 3% sulfuric acid in 95% ethanol (acid-alcohol) is the decolorizing agent, and methylene blue is the counterstain. Acid-fast organisms appear pink-red on a pale blue background. The contrast between organisms and background is sometimes poor, and fluorochrome stain is generally preferred for specimen examination. Acid-fast stains are used for detecting bacteria, including *Mycobacterium, Nocardia, Rhodococcus, Tsukamurella,* and *Gordona* spp., and the oocysts of *Cryptosporidium* spp., *Isospora belli, Sarcocystis* spp., and *Cyclospora* spp. Because some of these organisms lose the primary stain when they are exposed to 3% sulfuric acid, the decolorizing agent can be reduced to 0.5 to 1%. Organisms that retain this modified stain are referred to as being partially acid-fast.

Lugol's Iodine Stain

Iodine is added to wet preparations of parasitology specimens to enhance the contrast of the internal structures (e.g., nuclei, glycogen vacuoles). One disadvantage of this method is that protozoa are killed by the iodine and thus motility cannot be observed.

Methenamine Silver Stain

Methenamine silver staining is generally performed in surgical pathology laboratories rather than microbiology laboratories. It is primarily used for the detection of fungal elements in tissues, although other organisms (e.g., *Legionella* spp.) can be detected. Silver staining requires skill, because nonspecific staining can render the slide uninterpretable.

Methylene Blue Stain

Methylene blue is another contrasting dye commonly used in the laboratory, primarily for detection of bacteria and fungi. It can be mixed with potassium hydroxide and used to examine skin scrapings for fungal elements.

Periodic Acid-Schiff (PAS) Stain

Periodic acid-Schiff stain is used to detect yeast cells and fungal hyphae in tissues. Periodic acid (5%) hydrolyzes the cell wall aldehydes, which then combine with the modified Schiff reagent and stain the cell wall carbohydrates pink-magenta against a light green background. Because this staining procedure is complex, most laboratories have replaced it with the calcofluor white stain.

Potassium Hydroxide (KOH)

A 10 to 15% solution of potassium hydroxide can be used to dissolve cellular and organic debris and facilitate detection of fungal elements, which are not affected by strong alkali solutions (although fungal elements will dissolve after exposure for a few days). Ink (e.g., permanent blue-black Parker Super Quick Ink) can be added as a contrasting agent to aid in the detection of fungi.

Toluidine Blue-O Stain

Toluidine blue-O stain is used primarily for the detection of *Pneumocystis carinii* in respiratory specimens. The cysts of *Pneumocystis* stain reddish blue to dark purple on a light blue background. Trophozoites do not stain with this method. This staining method is rapid and inexpensive, but some skill is required to recognize *P. carinii* cysts (usually present in clumps). Many laboratories prefer the direct fluorescent-antibody test for detection of *P. carinii,* even though the stain is more expensive.

Trichrome Stain

Trichrome stain, like iron hematoxylin stain, is used for the detection and identification of protozoa. When staining is done properly, the specimen background is green and the protozoa have blue-green to purple cytoplasms with red or purple-red nuclei and inclusions.

Wright Stain

Wright stain is a polychromatic stain that contains a mixture of methylene blue, azure B (from the oxidation of methylene blue), and eosin Y dissolved in methanol. The eosin ions are negatively charged and stain the basic components of the cells orange to pink, while the other dyes stain the acidic cell structures various shades of blue to purple.

Ziehl-Neelsen Stain

Ziehl-Neelsen, an acid-fast stain, requires that the specimen be heated during staining so that the basic carbol fuchsin can penetrate into the organisms. Once this penetration is accomplished, decolorization and counterstaining are the same as with the Kinyoun method. The sensitivity and specificity of this stain are essentially the same as those of the Kinyoun method.

Specimen Processing

Table 4.3 Recommendations for primary stains and bacterial culture media

Type of specimen	Stain[a]		Culture medium[b]													
	Gram	AFB	BA	CHOC	MAC, EMB	TM, NYC	BLD-B	A-BA	BBE	LKV	A-CNA, A-PEA	THIO, CMB	XLD, HE	CAMPY	CIN	S-MAC
Abscess	R	O	×	×	×			×	×	×	×					
Catheter	N		×													
Ear																
External	O	N	×	×	×											
Internal	R	N	×	×	×							×				
Eye																
External	O	N	×	×												
Internal	R	N	×	×								×				
Fluids																
Amniotic	R	O	×	×	×		×	×	×	×	×					
Blood	N	N	×				×									
Bone marrow	R	O	×	×			×									
Cerebrospinal	R	O	×	×								×				
Culdocentesis	R	O	×	×	×		×	×	×	×	×					
Paracentesis (abdominal)	R	O	×	×	×		×	×	×	×	×					
Pericardial	R	O	×	×			×					×				
Pleural	R	O	×	×			×	×				×				
Synovial (joint)	R	O	×	×			×									

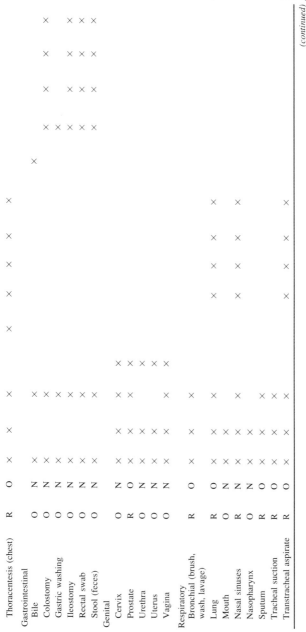

Specimen											
Thoracentesis (chest)	R	O	×				×			×	× × ×
Gastrointestinal											
Bile	O	N				×	×			×	× × ×
Colostomy	O	N	×			×	×			×	× × ×
Gastric washing	O	N	×			×	×	×		×	× × × ×
Ileostomy	O	N	×			×	×				
Rectal swab	O	N	×			×	×				
Stool (feces)	O	N	×			×	×			×	
Genital											
Cervix	O	N	×	×		×	×	×			
Prostate	R	O	×	×		×	×	×			
Urethra	O	N	×			×	×	×			
Uterus	O	N	×		×	×	×	×			
Vagina	O	N	×			×	×	×			
Respiratory											
Bronchial (brush, wash, lavage)	R	O	×			×	×				
Lung	R	O	×	×	×	×	×				
Mouth	O	N	×			×	×				
Nasal sinuses	R	N	×		×	×	×				
Nasopharynx	O	O	×			×					
Sputum	R	O	×		×	×	×				
Tracheal suction	R	O	×		×	×	×				
Transtracheal aspirate	R	O	×	×	×	×	×				

(continued)

Specimen Processing

Table 4.3 Recommendations for primary stains and bacterial culture media (*continued*)

	Stain[a]		Culture medium[b]												
Type of specimen	Gram	AFB	BA CHOC	MAC, TM, EMB NYC	BLD-B	A-BA	BBE	LKV	A-CNA, A-PEA	THIO, CMB	XLD, HE	CAMPY	CIN	S-MAC
Skin														
Superficial (e.g., cellulitis)	O	O	× ×	×										
Other (sinus tract, ulcer, fistula)	O	O	× ×	×										
Tissue														
Autopsy	O	O	× ×	×										
Burn	O	O	× ×	×										
Surgical	R	O	× ×	×		×	×	×	×					
Other (e.g., biopsy)	O	O	× ×	×		×	×	×	×					
Urine														
Catheterized	O		×	×										
Midstream voided	O		×	×										
Suprapubic aspirate	R		×	×	×									

[a] AFB, acid-fast bacillus; R, staining should be routinely performed; O, staining is optional and should be performed if requested; N, staining should not be performed unless the request is discussed with the physician.

[b] Abbreviations: BA, aerobic blood agar; CHOC, chocolate agar; MAC, MacConkey agar; EMB, eosin-methylene blue agar (either can be used); TM, NYC, Thayer-Martin agar and New York City agar (either can be used); BLD-B, blood culture bottle (used if more than 3 to 4 ml of fluid is received for processing); A-BA, anaerobic blood agar; BBE, *Bacteroides* bile esculin agar; LKV, kanamycin-vancomycin laked blood agar; A-CNA, A-PEA, anaerobic colistin-nalidixic agar and anaerobic phenylethyl alcohol agar (either can be used); THIO, CMB, thioglycolate broth and chopped-meat broth (either can be used); XLD, HE, xylose-lysine-deoxycholate agar and Hektoen enteric agar (either can be used); CAMPY, *Campylobacter* agar; CIN, cefsulodin-Irgasan-novobiocin agar; S-MAC, sorbitol-MacConkey agar.

Table 4.4 Recommendations for primary stains and fungal culture media

Type of specimen	Stain[a]		Culture medium[b]					
	KOH, CW	II	BHIA	BHIA-A, MYCO	IMA	BHIB	DTM
Abscess	R	N		×	×		
Catheter	N	N		×	×		
Ear	O	N		×	×		
Eye							
Corneal scraping	R	N		×	×	×	
Aspirate	R	N	×			×	
Fluids							
Blood	N	N	×				
Bone marrow	R	N	×		×		
Cerebrospinal	N	R	×			×	
Paracentesis	O	N	×		×		
Pleural	O	N	×		×		
Synovial	O	N	×		×		
Thoracentesis	O	N	×		×		

(continued)

Table 4.4 Recommendations for primary stains and fungal culture media *(continued)*

Type of specimen	Stain[a]		Culture medium[b]					
	KOH, CW	II	BHIA	BHIA-A, MYCO	IMA	BHIB	DTM	
Gastrointestinal								
Gastric washing	N	N		X	X			
Rectal swab	N	N		X	X			
Stool (feces)	N	N		X	X			
Genital								
Cervix	O	N		X	X			
Vagina	O	N		X	X			
Respiratory								
Bronchial (brush, wash, lavage)	O	O		X	X			
Lung	O	O		X	X			
Mouth	O	N		X	X			
Nasal sinuses	O	N		X	X	X		
Nasopharynx	O	N		X	X			

Specimen	KOH[a]	CW[a]	BHIA-A[b]	MYCO[b]	BHIB[b]	IMA[b]	DTM[b]
Sputum	O	O	X	X	X		
Tracheal suction	O	O	X	X	X		
Transtracheal aspirate	O	O	X	X	X		
Skin							
Hair	R	N	X	X		X	X
Nails	R	N	X	X		X	X
Skin scrapings	R	N	X	X		X	X
Tissue							
Autopsy	O	N	X	X	X		
Burn	O	N	X	X	X		
Surgical	O	O	X	X	X		
Urine	O	O	X				

---

[a] KOH, 10 to 15% potassium hydroxide with Parker Super Quick permanent black ink; CW, calcofluor white; II, India ink; R, staining should be routinely performed; O, staining is optional and should be performed if requested; N, staining should not be performed unless the request is discussed with the physician.

[b] BHIA, brain heart infusion agar with blood; BHIA-A, brain heart infusion agar supplemented with blood, gentamicin, chloramphenicol, and cycloheximide, and Mycosel or Mycobiotic agar (Sabouraud dextrose agar with cycloheximide and chloramphenicol) (one or more of these selective media can be used); IMA, inhibitory mold agar (with chloramphenicol); BHIB, brain heart infusion broth; DTM, dermatophyte test medium.

Specimen Processing: Virology

A large number of diverse viruses can be associated with common clinical symptoms (e.g., respiratory infection, exanthem). The table given here lists the most common viruses associated with each general symptom. Refer to Table 4.2 for guidance in the selection of a tissue culture cell line for the isolation of a particular virus. The Immunodiagnostic Tests section of this handbook lists common serologic tests that can be used to detect viral antigens and the antibodies directed against these viruses.

Table 4.5 Selection of clinical specimens for specific viral diseases

Clinical symptom(s)	Clinical specimens[a]	Common viruses
Upper respiratory tract infection	Nasopharyngeal swab, nasal washing, throat swab	Rhinovirus, influenza virus, parainfluenza virus, adenovirus, enterovirus, cytomegalovirus, Epstein-Barr virus, reovirus
Lower respiratory tract infection	Endotracheal aspirate, bronchial (washing, brushing, biopsy sample, lavage fluid), transtracheal aspirate, lung sample	Influenza virus, respiratory syncytial virus, parainfluenza virus, cytomegalovirus
Exanthems	Nasopharyngeal swab, throat swab, stool	Herpesvirus 6, parvovirus B19, enterovirus, rubeola virus, rubella virus
Vesicular lesions	Lesion swab, fluid, skin scraping	Herpes simplex virus, varicella-zoster virus, enterovirus

(continued)

Specimen Processing

Table 4.5 Selection of clinical specimens for specific viral diseases *(continued)*

Clinical symptom(s)	Clinical specimens[a]	Common viruses
Central nervous system disease	CSF, nasopharyngeal swab, brain, (stool)	Enterovirus, herpesviruses, arboviruses
Enteritis and diarrhea	Stool, colon sample	Rotavirus, enteric adenovirus, astrovirus, calicivirus
Congenital anomalies	Nasopharyngeal swab, urine, blood, tissue from diseased organs	Cytomegalovirus, herpes simplex virus, rubella virus, varicella-zoster virus
Posttransplantation syndromes	Throat swab, blood, buffy coat cells, transplanted organ, (urine)	Herpes simplex virus, cytomegalovirus, Epstein-Barr virus, herpesvirus 6

[a] CSF, cerebrospinal fluid. Parentheses indicate specimens that are usable but not preferred.
Source: D. A. Lennette, p. 869, *in* P. R. Murray, E. J. Baron, M. A. Pfaller, F. C. Tenover, and R. H. Yolken. *Manual of Clinical Microbiology,* 6th ed., American Society for Microbiology, Washington, D.C., 1995.

Specimen Processing: Parasitology

Most parasites are detected by microscopic examination of clinical specimens. The table that follows lists specimens, the most commonly observed parasites, and the methods used to detect them.

Specimen Processing

Table 4.6 Detection of the most common parasites in clinical specimens

Specimen	Parasite	Diagnostic method[a]						
		Wet mount	Permanent stain	Giemsa stain	Acid-fast stain	DFA stain	H&E stain	Culture
Feces	Amebae	×	×			×		
	Ciliates	×	×					
	Flagellates	×	×					
	Coccidia				×	×		
	Microsporidia		×		×	×		
	Cestodes	×						
	Nematodes	×						
	Trematodes	×						
Intestinal biopsy sample	*Entamoeba histolytica*		×	×				
	Giardia lamblia		×	×				
	Coccidia				×	×		
	Microsporidia		×	×	×	×		

Specimen	Organism	1	2	3	4	5	6
Blood, buffy coat cells	*Babesia* spp.						×
	Plasmodium spp.		×				×
	Leishmania spp.		×				
	Trypanosomes		×				
	Microfilariae		×				
Bone marrow	*Leishmania* spp.		×				×
Lung	*Toxoplasma* spp.		×			×	×
	Entamoeba histolytica	×	×				
Liver	*Entamoeba histolytica*	×	×				
	Cryptosporidium spp.		×		×		
	Microsporidia				×	×	
	Toxoplasma spp.		×				×
	Leishmania spp.	×	×				
	Echinococcus spp.			×			
Brain	*Acanthamoeba* spp.		×				×
	Naegleria spp.		×				×
	Balamuthia spp.	×	×				×
	Toxoplasma spp.		×			×	×

(continued)

Specimen Processing

Table 4.6 Detection of the most common parasites in clinical specimens *(continued)*

Specimen	Parasite	Diagnostic method[a]						
		Wet mount	Permanent stain	Giemsa stain	Acid-fast stain	DFA stain	H&E stain	Culture
Eye	*Acanthamoeba* spp.		×	×				×
	Microsporidia		×	×	×			
Skin	*Leishmania* spp.			×				×
	Onchocerca spp.			×			×	
	Mansonella spp.			×			×	
Muscle	Trypanosomes			×				×
	Trichinella spp.	×						
Lymph nodes	*Leishmania* spp.			×				×
	Trypanosomes			×				×

[a] DFA, direct fluorescent antibody; H&E, hematoxylin and eosin.

Identification of microbes is a major function of the clinical microbiology laboratory. The identity of an organism can be used to assess its medical importance, determine its site of origin, and guide empiric antimicrobial therapy. The following section details in tabular format the identification of common bacteria, yeasts, and parasites. This section is intended to serve as a guide to microbial identification; the user can find more extensive identification schemes in the *Manual of Clinical Microbiology,* 6th ed. (1995), *Clinical Microbiology Procedures Handbook* (1992), and Baron's *Diagnostic Microbiology* (1994). Identification of molds, which is too complex to be discussed comprehensively in this book, is primarily determined by morphological parameters. Please refer to one of the texts cited above or to Larone's *Medically Important Fungi: a Guide to Identification* (1995). Virus identification is also not discussed here, because viral identifications are determined by growth of the viruses in specific eukaryotic cells and immunologic testing. This information is presented in Sections 4 and 7.

The symbols used throughout this section are explained here.

Test reactivity: 0, <10% of the tests are positive; +, >90% of the tests are positive; V, test reactions are variable; W, positive tests are weak and develop slowly; NT, organism was not tested in the specific reaction; S, the organism is susceptible to the antibiotic or reagent; R, the organism is resistant to the antibiotic or reagent. Superscript designations mean that the indicated reaction is atypical but does occur with specific strains or species. Parentheses indicate that the positive reaction develops slowly. Metabolic products (GLC): A, acetic acid; B, butyric acid; C, caproic acid; IB, isobutyric acid; IC, isocaproic acid; IV, isovaleric acid; L, lactic acid; P, propionic acid; PA, phenylacetic acid; S, succinic acid; V, valeric acid. Capital letters indicate a major acid peak, lowercase letters indicate a minor peak, and parentheses indicate acids irregularly observed.

Bacteriology

See Tables 5.1 to 5.33 and Flowchart 5.1.

Table 5.1 Differential characteristics of gram-positive cocci and coccobacilli

Genus	Cell arrangement[a]	Type of colony[b]	Hemolysis[c]	Motility	Atmosphere[d]	6.5% NaCl	10°C	45°C	Furazolidone (100 µg)	Lysostaphin (200 µg)	Vancomycin (30 µg)	Catalase	Oxidase	PYR[e]	Leucine aminopeptidase	Bile-esculin	Gas from glucose
						Growth properties						Biochemical reactions					
Abiotrophia	Ch, Pr	0	A	0	F	0	0	0	S	NT	S	0	0	+	+	0	0
Aerococcus	T, Pr	0	A	0	F	+	0	+	S	R	S	0[w]	0	v	v	v	0
Alloiococcus	Cb, Pr, T	0	A	NT	Ae	+	NT	NT	S	NT	S	+[w]	0	+	+	NT	NT
Enterococcus	Ch, Pr	0	A, B, N	0[v]	F	+	NT	+	S	R	S[R]	0	0	+	+	+	0
Gemella	Pr	0	A, N	0	F	0	0	0	S	NT	S	0	0	+	v	0	0
Globicatella	Ch, Ch, Pr	0	A	0	F	+	0	0	S	NT	S	0	0	+	0	0	0
Helcococcus	Pr, Cl	0	N	0	F	+	0	0	S	NT	S	0	0	+	0	+	0
Lactobacillus	Ch, Cb	0	N	0	F	v	v	v	S	NT	R	0	0	0	v	v	v
Lactococcus	Ch, Cb, Pr	0	A, N	0	F	v	+	0[v]	S	NT	S	0	0	v	+	+[v]	0
Leuconostoc	Ch, Ch, Pr	0	A, N	0	F	v	+	v	S	NT	R	0	0	0	0	v	+

(continued)

Microbial Identification

Table 5.1 Differential characteristics of gram-positive cocci and coccobacilli (*continued*)

Genus	Cell arrangement[a]	Type of colony[b]	Hemolysis[c]	Motility	Atmosphere[d]	Growth properties						Biochemical reactions					
						6.5% NaCl	10°C	45°C	Furazolidone (100 µg)	Lysostaphin (200 µg)	Vancomycin (30 µg)	Catalase	Oxidase	PYR[e]	Leucine aminopeptidase	Bile-esculin	Gas from glucose
Micrococcus	Cl, T	A, P	N	0	Ae	+	V	V	R	R	S	+	+	0	NT	$+^v$	0
Pediococcus	T, Pr	0	A	0	F	V	0	+	S	NT	R	0	0	0	+	$+^v$	0
Planococcus	T, Pr	P	N	+	Ae	+	NT	NT	S	R	S	0	0	0	NT	NT	0
Staphylococcus	Cl	P	A, B, N	0	F	+	V	V	S	S	S	+	0	0	NT	V	0
Stomatococcus	Ch, Pr	A	N	0	F	0	0	0	V	R	S	V	0	+	+	0	0
Streptococcus	Ch, Pr	0	A, B, N	0	F	0^v	0	V	S	R	S	0	0	0^+	+	0^v	0
Tetragenococcus	Cl, T	0	A	0	F	+	0	+	S	NT	S	0	0	0	+	+	0
Vagococcus	Cb, Ch	0	A, N	+	F	+	+	0	S	NT	S	0	0	+	+	+	0

[a] Cb, coccobacillus; Ch, chains; Cl clusters; Pr, pairs; T, tetrad.
[b] A, adherent; P, pigmented.
[c] A, alpha; B, beta; N, nonhemolytic.
[d] Ae, aerobic; F, facultatively anaerobic.
[e] PYR, pyrrolidonyl arylamidase.

Table 5.2 Catalase reactivity

Positive reactivity	Negative reactivity		
Aerococcus	*Abiotrophia*	*Helcococcus*	*Planococcus*
Alloiococcus	*Aerococcus*	*Lactobacillus*	*Stomatococcus*
Micrococcus	*Alloiococcus*	*Lactococcus*	*Streptococcus*
Staphylococcus	*Enterococcus*	*Leuconostoc*	*Tetragenococcus*
Stomatococcus	*Gemella*	*Pediococcus*	*Vagococcus*
	Globicatella		

Table 5.3 Vancomycin susceptibility

Susceptibility			Resistance
Abiotrophia	*Helcococcus*	*Streptococcus*	*Enterococcus*
Aerococcus	*Lactococcus*	*Tetragenococcus*	*Lactobacillus*
Alloiococcus	*Micrococcus*	*Vagococcus*	*Leuconostoc*
Enterococcus	*Planococcus*		*Pediococcus*
Gemella	*Staphylococcus*		
Globicatella	*Stomatococcus*		

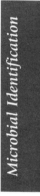

Microbial Identification

Table 5.4 Pyrrolidonyl arylamidase reactivity

PYR^a positive		PYR negative	
Abiotrophia	*Helcococcus*	*Aerococcus*	*Pediococcus*
Aerococcus	*Lactococcus*	*Lactobacillus*	*Planococcus*
Alloiococcus	*Stomatococcus*	*Lactococcus*	*Staphylococcus*
Enterococcus	*Streptococcus*	*Leuconostoc*	*Streptococcus*
Gemella	*Vagococcus*	*Micrococcus*	*Tetragenococcus*
Globicatella			

^a PYR, pyrrolidonyl arylamidase.

Table 5.5   Leucine aminopeptidase production

Genera			
LAP[a] positive		**LAP negative**	
Abiotrophia	*Lactococcus*	*Aerococcus*	*Helcococcus*
Aerococcus	*Pediococcus*	*Gemella*	*Lactobacillus*
Alloiococcus	*Stomatococcus*	*Globicatella*	*Leuconostoc*
Enterococcus	*Streptococcus*		
Gemella	*Tetragenococcus*		
Lactobacillus	*Vagococcus*		

[a] LAP, leucine aminopeptidase.

Table 5.6 Differential characteristics of common *Staphylococcus* species

Staphylococcus species	Colony pigment	Coagulase	Clumping factor	Acid from: Cellobiose	Maltose	Mannitol	Mannose	Sucrose	Trehalose	Turanose	Xylose	Heat-stable nuclease	Alkaline phosphatase	PYR[a]	Ornithine decarboxylase	Urease	β-Galactosidase	Acetoin production[b]	Novobiocin	Polymyxin B
S. aureus	+	+	+	o	+	+	+	+	+	+	o	+	+	o	o	V	o	+	S	R
S. epidermidis	o	o	o	o	+	o	+	+	o	V	o	o	+	o	V	+	o	+	S	R
S. haemolyticus	V	o	o	o	+	V	o	+	+	V	o	o	o	+	o	o	o	+	S	S
S. hyicus	o	V	o	o	o	o	+	+	+	o	o	+	+	o	o	V	o	o	S	R
S. intermedius	o	+	V	o	V	V	+	+	+	V	o	+	+	+	o	+	+	o	S	S
S. lugdunensis	V	o	+	o	+	o	+	+	+	V	o	o	o	+	+	V	o	+	S	V
S. saprophyticus	V	o	o	o	+	V	o	+	+	+	o	o	o	o	o	+	+	+	R	S
S. schleiferi	o	o	+	o	o	o	+	o	V	o	o	+	+	+	o	o	V	+	S	S

[a] PYR, pyrrolidonyl arylamidase.
[b] In Voges-Proskauer test.

Flowchart 5.1 Preliminary differentiation of selected gram-positive cocci

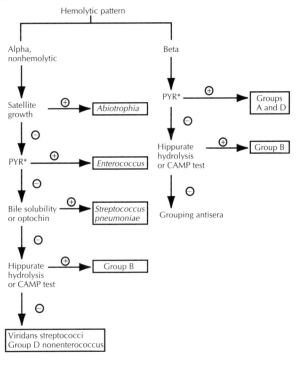

*PYR, Pyrrolidonyl arylamidase

Table 5.7 Differential properties of viridans group streptococci

Streptococcus species and group	Mannitol	Sorbitol	Voges-Proskauer	Arginine hydrolysis	Esculin hydrolysis	Group D	PYR[a]	Urease
S. mutans group (includes S. mutans, S. rattus, and S. cricetus)	+	+	+	0[b]	+	0	0	0
S. salivarius group (includes S. salivarius and S. vestibularius)[c]	0	0	+[d]	0	+	0	0	V
S. sanguis group (includes S. sanguis, S. gordonii, S. crista, and S. parasanguis)	0	0	0	+[e]	+[f]	0	0	0

(continued)

Microbial Identification

Table 5.7 Differential properties of viridans group streptococci *(continued)*

Streptococcus species and group	Mannitol	Sorbitol	Voges-Proskauer	Arginine hydrolysis	Esculin hydrolysis	Group D	PYR[a]	Urease
S. mitis (includes *S. mitior*, *S. oralis*, and *S. sanguis* II)	0	0	0	0	0	0	0	0
S. milleri group (includes *S. intermedius*, *S. constellatus*, and *S. anginosus*)	V	0	+	+	V	0	0	0
S. bovis[c]	V[g]	0	+	0	+	+	0	0

[a] PYR, pyrrolidonyl arylamidase.
[b] *S. rattus* is arginine positive.
[c] The urease test differentiates *S. salivarius* (about 70% positive) from mannitol-negative strains of *S. bovis*.
[d] *S. vestibularius* is Voges-Proskauer variable.
[e] *S. crista* may be arginine dihydrolase negative.
[f] *S. crista* is esculin negative; *S. parasanguis* may be esculin negative.
[g] *S. bovis* biotype I is positive; biotype II is negative.

Table 5.8 Differential characteristics of *Enterococcus* species

Group	Enterococcus species	Motility (30°C)	Yellow pigment	Arginine dihydrolase	Acid from: Mannitol	Sorbitol	Arabinose	Raffinose	Sucrose	Pyruvate
I	*E. avium*	0	0	0	+	+	+	0	+	+
	E. malodoratus	0	0	0	+	+	0	+	+	+
	E. raffinosus	0	0	0	+	+	+	+	+	+
	E. pseudoavium	0	0	0	+	+	0	0	+	+
II	*E. faecalis*	0	0	+	+	+	0	0	$+^0$	+
	E. faecium	0	0	+	+	0^+	+	0^+	$+^0$	0
	E. casseliflavus	+	+	+	+	0^+	+	+	+	0^+
	E. mundtii	0	+	+	+	0^+	+	+	+	0
	E. gallinarum	+	0	+	+	0	+	+	+	0
III	*E. durans*	0	0	+	0	0	0	0	0	0
	E. hirae	0	0	+	0	0	0	+	+	0
	E. dispar	0	0	+	0	0	0	+	+	+
	E. faecalis (variant)	0	0	+	0	0	0	0	0	+

Microbial Identification

Microbial Identification

Table 5.9 Differential characteristics of anaerobic, gram-positive cocci[a]

Peptostreptococcus species	Indole	Nitrate reductase	Alkaline phosphatase	Urease	SPS	Glucose fermentation	Metabolic products (GLC)
P. anaerobius	0	0	0	0	S	W	A, IC, ib, b, iv
P. asaccharolyticus	+	0	0	0	R	0	A, B
P. magnus	0	0	0	0	R	0	A
P. micros	0	0	+	0	R	0	A
P. prevotii	0	V	0	+	R	W	B, C, iv, a
P. hydrogenalis	+	0	+	0	R	+	B, a, p, l
P. indolicus	+	+	0	0	R	0	A, B, p
P. tetradius	0	0	0	+	R	+	B, L
P. productus	0	0	0	0	R	+	A

[a] The most common clinical isolates from human specimens are P. anaerobius (large cocci or coccobacilli in pairs and chains and large colonies with a sweet odor [isocaproic acid]), P. asaccharolyticus (cocci in pairs, tetrads, and clumps), P. magnus (large cocci in tetrads), P. micros (small cocci in pairs and chains), and P. prevotii (cocci in pairs and tetrads). SPS, sodium polyanethol sulfonate; GLC, gas-liquid chromatography.

Table 5.10 Differential characteristics of gram-positive coryneform bacilli

Type of bacillus and genera[a]	Motility	Nitrate reductase	Urease	Hydrolysis		Acid from:					
				Esculin	Gelatin	Glucose	Xylose	Mannose	Maltose	Lactose	Sucrose
Catalase-negative											
Archanobacterium	0	0	0	0	0	+	0	0	+	+	V
Erysipelothrix	0	0	0	0	0	V	0	0	0	+	0
Gardnerella	0	0	0	0	0	+	V	V	+	V	V
Catalase-positive, fermentative											
Corynebacterium	0	V	V	0	0	$+^0$	0	0	$+^0$	0	V
Dermabacter	0	0	0	+	0	+	V	0	+	+	+
Listeria	+	0	0	+	0	+	0	0	NT	NT	NT
Catalase-positive, nonfermentative											
Brevibacterium	0	0^+	0	0	+	0	0	0	0	0	0
Turicella	0	0	0	0	NT	0	0	0	0	0	0

[a] *Archanobacterium haemolyticum* produces pinpoint, beta-hemolytic colonies with a positive CAMP test; *Erysipelothrix rhusiopathiae* is a thin, short, or filamentous bacillus that produces H$_2$S on triple sugar iron slants; *Gardnerella vaginalis* is a gram-variable to gram-negative bacillus that is hemolytic on human blood agar; *Corynebacterium* spp. are very heterogeneous; *Dermabacter hominis* is a coccoid bacterium found on the skin; *Listeria monocytogenes* is a coccobacillus that appears in pairs and short chains, has weakly hemolytic colonies on sheep blood, and is hippurate and Voges-Proskauer positive; *Brevibacterium* spp. are coccoid bacteria found in food and on the skin; *Turicella otitidis* is a branching, pleomorphic bacillus that is CAMP positive and is associated with ear infections.

Microbial Identification

Microbial Identification

Table 5.11 Differential characteristics of selected *Corynebacterium* species

Corynebacterium species	Nitrate reductase	Urease	Pyrazinamidase	Phospholipase D	Alkaline phosphatase	Acid from:			
						Glucose	Maltose	Ribose	Sucrose
C. diphtheriae subsp. *mitis*	+	0	0	0	0	+	+	V	0
C. diphtheriae subsp. *gravis*	+	0	0	0	0	+	+	+	0
C. diphtheriae subsp. *intermedius*	+	0	0	0	0	+	+	+	0
C. jeikeium	0	0	+	0	+	+	V	+	0
C. minutissimum	0	0	+	NT	+	+	+	V	V
C. pseudodiphtheriticum	+	+	+	0	0	0	0	0	0
C. striatum	+	0	+	NT	+	+	0	V	+
C. ulcerans	0	+	0	+	+	+	+	+	0
C. urealyticum	0	+	+	NT	V	0	0	0	0
C. xerosis	V	0[+]	+[0]	0	+[0]	+	V	+	+

Table 5.12 Differential characteristics of selected *Bacillus* species

Bacillus species	Catalase	Spores[a]	Penicillin	Citrate utilization	Tyrosine hydrolysis	Growth in 7% NaCl	Voges-Proskauer reaction	Lecithinase	Growth at: 50°C	Growth at: 60°C	Acid from: Glucose	Acid from: Arabinose	Acid from: Xylose	Acid from: Mannitol
B. anthracis[b]	+	OC	S	0[+]	0	+	+	+	0	0	+	0	0	0
B. cereus	+	OC	R	+	+	+	+	+	0	0	+	0	0	0
B. licheniformis	+	OC	S	+	0	+	+	0	+	0	+	+	+	+
B. stearothermophilus	>	OT	NT	0	0	0	0	0	+	+	+	>	>	>
B. subtilis	+	OC	S	+	0	+	+	0	>	0	+	+	+	+

[a] O, oval; C, central; T, terminal or subterminal.
[b] *B. anthracis* is nonmotile and nonhemolytic and forms a capsule.

Microbial Identification

Microbial Identification

Table 5.13 Differential characteristics of non-acid-fast actinomycetes

Actinomycete genus[a]	Lysozyme (0.05%)	Ethylene glycol degradation	Growth on paraffin	Anaerobic growth	Nitrate reductase	Urease	Motility	Casein	Hypoxanthine	Tyrosine	Xanthine	Gelatin
								Hydrolysis of:				
Actinomadura	S	0	0	0	+	0	0	+	+	+	0	+
Dermatophilus	S	0	0	+	0	+	+	NT	NT	NT	NT	NT
Nocardiopsis	S	0	0	0	+	+	0	+	+	+	+	+
Oerskovia	S	0	0	+	+°	V	+°	+	V	0	V	+
Streptomyces	S	0	0	0	+°	+°	+°	+	+	+	+°	V

[a] *Actinomadura* colonies are leathery red with short aerial hyphae; *Dermatophilus* colonies are yellow, orange, or gray with short aerial hyphae; *Nocardiopsis* colonies are brownish red with abundant aerial hyphae; *Oerskovia* colonies are bright yellow with no aerial hyphae; *Streptomyces* colonies are chalky white or colored with short aerial hyphae.

Table 5.14 Differential characteristics of partially acid-fast bacilli

Species	Cell morphology[a]	Growth at 45°C	Catalase	Hydrolysis of: Casein	Hydrolysis of: Hypoxanthine	Hydrolysis of: Tyrosine	Hydrolysis of: Xanthine	Hydrolysis of: Gelatin	Hydrolysis of: Starch	Acid from: Glucose	Acid from: Rhamnose	Nitrate reductase	Urease	Arylsulfatase[b]	Lysozyme (0.05%)
Nocardia asteroides complex															
N. asteroides	B, CB, H	$+^{0}$	+	0	0	0	0	0	0	+	0^{+}	+	+	0	R
N. farcinica	B, CB, H	+	+	0	0	0	0	0	0	+	$+^{0}$	+	+	0	R
N. nova	B, CB, H	0	+	0	0^{0}	0	0	0	0	+	0	+	+	+	R
Nocardia brasiliensis	B, CB, H	0^{0}	+	+	+	+	0	+	0	+	0	+	+	0	R
Nocardia otitidiscaviarum	B, CB, H	$+^{0}$	+	0	+	0	+	0	0	+	0	+	+	0	R
Nocardia transvalensis	B, CB, H	0	+	0^{+}	$+^{0}$	0^{+}	$+^{0}$	0	+	+	0	$+^{0}$	+	0	R^{S}
Rhodococcus equi	B, CB	NT	+	0	0	0^{0}	0	0	0^{0}	0	0	$+^{0}$	$+^{0}$	0	R^{S}
Rhodococcus spp.	B, CB	NT	+	0	0	0^{+}	0	+	NT	V	V	+	+	0	S
Gordona spp.	C, CB	NT	+	0	0	0	0	0	NT	NT	NT	+	+	0	S
Tsukamurella spp.	C, CB	NT	+	0	+	0	+	+	NT	NT	NT	0	+	0	R

[a] B, bacilli; C, cocci; CB, coccobacilli; H, hyphal forms.
[b] After 14 days.

Microbial Identification

Table 5.15 Differential characteristics of nonchromogenic, slow-growing mycobacteria

Mycobacterium species	Colony morphology[a]	Niacin	Nitrate reductase	Catalase (>45 mm)	Tween 80 hydrolysis	Urease	Arylsulfatase[b]	Growth On T2H[c]	On PZA[d]	In 5% NaCl
M. tuberculosis	R	+	+	0	V	V	0	+	+	0
M. africanum	R	0	0	0	0	+	0	V	0	0
M. bovis	R	0	0	0	0	V	0	0	0	0
M. siniae[e]	S	V	0	+	0	+	0	+	+	0
M. avium complex	S	0	0	0	0	0	0	+	+	0
M. xenopi	S	0	0	+	0	0	V	+	V	0
M. haemophilum	R	0	0	0	0	0	0	+	+	0
M. malmoense	S	0	0	0	+	0	0	+	+	0
M. shimoidei	R	0	0	0	+	0	0	+	+	0
M. genavense	S	0	0	+	+	+	0	+	+	NT
M. celatum	S	0	0	0	0	0	+	+	+	0
M. ulcerans	R	0	0	0	0	V	0	+	0	0
M. terrae complex	S/R	0	0	+	+	V	0	+	V	0
M. triviale	R	0	0	+	+	V	V	+	V	+
M. gastri	S/R	0	0	0	+	V	0	+	0	0
M. nonchromogenicum	S/R	0	0	+	+	0	0	+	V	0

[a] R, rough; S, smooth. [b] After 3 days. [c] T2H, thiophene-2-carboxylic acid hydrazide. [d] PZA, pyrazinamidase. [e] Most strains are chromogenic.

Table 5.16 Differential characteristics of chromogenic, slow-growing mycobacteria

Mycobacterium species	Pigmentation[a]	Rapid growth at 30°C	Niacin production	Nitrate reductase	Catalase (>45 mm)	Tween 80 hydrolysis	Urease	Arylsulfatase[b]	Growth in 5% NaCl
M. kansasii	P	0	0	+	+	+	V	0	0
M. marinum	P	+	0	0	0	+	+	V	0
M. simiae	P[N]	0	V	0	+	0	V	0	0
M. asiaticum	P	0	0	0	+	+	0	0	0
M. szulgae	P (25°C) S (37°C)	0	0	+	+	V	+	0	0
M. gordonae	S	0	0	0	+	+	V	0	0
M. scrofulaceum	S	0	0	0	+	0	V	0	0
M. flavescens	S	0	0	+	+	+	V	0	V
M. xenopi	N[S]	0	0	0	+	0	0	V	0
M. avium complex	N[S]	0	0	0	0	0	0	0	0

[a] P, photochromogen; S, scotochromogen; N, nonchromogenic.
[b] After 3 days.

Microbial Identification

Microbial Identification

Table 5.17 Differential characteristics of rapidly growing mycobacteria

Mycobacterium species	Growth on MAC[a]	Nitrate reductase	Catalase (>45 mm)	68°C catalase	Tween 80 hydrolysis	Arylsulfatase[b]	Growth in 5% NaCl	Iron uptake	Sodium citrate	Inositol	Mannitol
M. fortuitum	+	+	+	+	V	+	+	+	0	0	0
M. abscessus	+	0	+	V	V	+	+	0	0	0	0
M. chelonae	+	0	+	V	V	+	0	0	+	0	0
M. chelonae-like organisms	V	V	0	V	0	V	0	V	+	0	+
M. peregrinum	+	+	+	NT	V	+	+	+	0	0	+
M. smegmatis	+	+	+	+	+	0	+	+	V	+	+
M. phlei	0	+	+	+	+	0	+	+	0	0	+
M. vaccae	0	+	+	+	+	0	V	+	+	NT	+
M. fallax	0	+	V	0	NT	0	0	0	0	0	0

[a] MAC, MacConkey agar.
[b] After 3 days.

Table 5.18 Differential characteristics of non-spore-forming, gram-positive anaerobic bacilli

Genus	Strict anaerobe	Motility	Catalase	Indole production	Nitrate reductase	Metabolic products (GLC)[a]
Actinomyces	V	0	V	0	V	S, L, a
Bifidobacterium	+	0	0	0	0	A, L
Eubacterium	+	V	0	0	V	a, b
Lactobacillus	V	0	0	0	0	L, (a), (s)
Mobiluncus	+	+	0	0	V	S, L, A
Propionibacterium	V	0	V	0	V	A, P, iv, s, l
Rothia	0	0	+	0	+	A, L, (s), (p)

[a] GLC, gas-liquid chromatography.

Microbial Identification

Table 5.19 Differential characteristics of selected *Actinomyces* and *Propionibacterium* spp.

Species	Catalase	Nitrate reductase	Indole	Urease	Esculin	Gelatin	Glucose	Arabinose	Mannose	Raffinose	Trehalose	Inositol	Glycerol	Xylose	Mannitol	Metabolic products (GLC)[a]
					Hydrolysis		Acid from:									
A. israelii	0	V	0	0	+	0	+	+	+	+	(+)	+	0	+	(+)	A, L, S
A. meyeri	0	0	0	0	V	0	+	0	0	0	0	0	(+)	+	0	A, S
A. naeslundii	0	+	0	+°	+	0	+	0	0	0	(+)	+	(+)	(+)	0	A, L, S
A. odontolyticus	0	V	0	0	V	0	+	0	0	0	0	0	(+)	(+)	0	A, S
A. pyogenes	0	0	0	0	0	+	+	0	(+)	0	(+)	(+)	0	(+)	0	A, S
A. viscosus	+	V	0	V	+	0	+	0	0	+	V	(+)	(+)	0	0	A, L, S
P. acnes	+	+	+°	0	0	+	+	0	+	0	0	0	+°	0	+°	A, P, (iv, l, s)
P. propionicus	0	+	0	0	0	V	+	0	(+)	+	(+)	(+)	(+)	0	(+)	A, P, (l, s)

[a] GLC, gas-liquid chromatography.

Table 5.20 Differential characteristics of selected *Clostridium* spp.

Clostridium species[a]	Spores[b]	Gelatin hydrolysis	Milk digestion	Lipase	Lecithinase	Indole	Nitrate reductase	Esculin hydrolysis	Acid from: Glucose	Maltose	Lactose	Sucrose	Salicin	Mannitol	Metabolic products (GLC)[c]
Saccharolytic, proteolytic															
C. bifermentans	OS	+	+	0	+	+	0	+	+	+[0]	0	0	0	0	A, (p, ib, b, iv, ic, s)
C. botulinum group I	OS	+	+	+	0	0	0	+	+	0[+]	0	0	0	0	A, B, IV, (p, ib, v, ic)
C. botulinum group II	OS	+	+	+	V	V	0	+	+	V	0	0	0	0	A, P, B, (v)
C. cadaveris	OT	+	+	0	0	+	0	0	+	0	0	0	0[+]	0	A, B, (p)
C. difficile	OS	+	0	0	0	0	0	+	+	0	0	0	0[+]	V	A, B, (p, ib, iv, v, ic)

(*continued*)

Microbial Identification

Table 5.20 Differential characteristics of selected *Clostridium* spp. *(continued)*

Clostridium species[a]	Spores[b]	Gelatin hydrolysis	Milk digestion	Lipase	Lecithinase	Indole	Nitrate reductase	Esculin hydrolysis	Acid from: Glucose	Maltose	Lactose	Sucrose	Salicin	Mannitol	Metabolic products (GLC)[c]
C. novyi type A	OS	+	0	+	+	0	0	0	+	V	0	0	V	0	A, P, B
C. novyi type B	OS	+	+	0	+	V	0	0	+	V	0	0	0	0	A, P, B
C. perfringens	OS	+	+	0	+	0	$+^{\circ}$	0	+	+	+	+	0	0	A, B, (p)
C. putrificum	OT	+	+	0	0	0	0	0	+	0	0	0	0	0	A, B, (ib, iv, p, ic, v, s)
C. septicum	OS	+	+	0	0	0	V	+	+	+	+	0	V	0	A, B, (p)
C. sordellii	OS	+	+	0	+	+	0	0	+	V	0	0	0	0	A, (p, ib, iv, ic)
C. sporogenes	OS	+	+	+	0	0	0	+	+	V	0	0	0	0	A, B, (p, ib, iv, ic, v)

Saccharolytic, nonproteolytic													
C. botulinum group III	OS	+	0	0	0	+	+	+	0	+	0	0	A, B
C. butyricum	OS	0	0	0	0	+	+	+	+	+	+	V	A, B
C. clostridioforme	OS	0	0	0	V	+°	+	+	+	V	V	0	A
C. innocuum	OT	0	0	0	0	0	+	+	0	+	+	+	A, B
C. ramosum	R/OT	0	0	0	0	0	+	+	+	+	+	V	A
C. tertium	OT	0	0	0	0	0	+	+	+	+	+	+	A, B
Asaccharolytic, proteolytic													
C. histolyticum	OS	+	0	0	0	0	0	0	0	0	0	0	A
C. limosum	OS	+	0	+	0	+	0	0	0	0	0	0	A
C. subterminale	OS	+	0	V	0	V	0	0	0	0	0	0	A, B, IV, (p, ib, ic)
C. tetani	RT	+	V	0	V	0	0	0	0	0	0	0	A, B, (p)

[a] Species commonly gram negative: *C. clostridioforme* and *C. ramosum*; aerotolerant species: *C. histolyticum* and *C. tertium*; nonmotile species: *C. innocuum*, *C. perfringens*, and *C. ramosum*; urease-positive species: *C. sordellii*.
[b] O, oval; R, round; T, terminal; S, subterminal. Spores are seldom observed for *C. clostridioforme*, *C. perfringens*, *C. ramosum*, and *C. subterminale*.
[c] GLC, gas-liquid chromatography.

Microbial Identification

Microbial Identification

Table 5.21 Differential characteristics of selected oxidase-positive, gram-negative cocci and coccobacilli

Genus and species	Growth: MacConkey	Growth: Modified Thayer-Martin	Growth: 42°C	Motility	Indole production	Catalase	Urease	Nitrate reductase	Phenylalanine deaminase	Gelatin hydrolysis	Acid from: Glucose	Maltose	Lactose	Sucrose	Fructose
Moraxella catarrhalis	0	>	0	0	0	+	0	+	0	0	0	0	0	0	0
Moraxella lacunata	0	0	0	0	0	+	0	+	>	>	0	0	0	0	0
Moraxella nonliquefaciens	0	0	>	0	0	+	0	+	0	0	0	0	0	0	0
Moraxella osloensis	>	0	>	>	0	+	0	>	0	0	0	0	0	0	0
Oligella ureolytica	>	0	0	>	0	+	+	+	+	0	0	0	0	0	0
Oligella urethralis	>	0	+	0	0	+	0	0	+	0	0	0	0	0	0
Neisseria gonorrhoeae	0	+	0	0	NT	+	NT	0	NT	NT	+	0	0	0	0
Neisseria meningitidis	0	+	0	0	NT	+	NT	0	NT	NT	+	+	0	0	0

Table 5.22 Differential characteristics of *Haemophilus* species

Haemophilus species[a]	Growth requirement			Hemolysis (horse blood)	Catalase	Acid from:				
	CO_2[b]	Hemin (X factor)	NAD (V factor)			Glucose	Sucrose	Lactose	Mannose	
H. aphrophilus	+	0	0	0	0	+	+	+	+	
H. ducreyi	0	+	0	0	0	0	0	0	0	
H. haemolyticus	0	+	+	+	+	+	0	0	0	
H. influenzae	+	+	+	0	+	+	0	0	0	
H. parahaemolyticus	0	0	+	+	+	+	+	0	0	
H. parainfluenzae	V	0	+	0	V	+	+	0	+	
H. paraphrophilus	+	0	+	0	0	+	+	+	+	
H. segnis	0	0	+	0	V	W	W	0	0	

[a] Indole production, urease, and ornithine decarboxylase reactions are used to differentiate *H. influenzae* and *H. parainfluenzae* biotypes.
[b] CO_2 enhances growth.

Microbial Identification

Microbial Identification

Table 5.23 Differential characteristics of selected species of the family *Enterobacteriaceae*

Species	Indole	Methyl red	Voges-Proskauer	Citrate	Urease	Phenylalanine deaminase	Lysine decarboxylase	Arginine dihydrolase	Ornithine decarboxylase	Motility (36°C)	Acid from: Glucose	Acid from: Lactose
Citrobacter spp.												
C. (diversus) koseri	+	+	0	+	V	0	0	+°	+	+	+	V
C. freundii	V	+	0	V	V	0	0	V	0	+°	+	+°
Edwardsiella tarda	+	+	0	0	0	0	+	0	+	+	+	0
Enterobacter spp.												
E. aerogenes	0	0	+	+	0	0	+	0	+	+	+	+
E. cloacae	0	0	+	+	V	0	0	+	+	+	+	+
Escherichia coli	+	+	0	0	0	0	+	0⁺	V	+	+	+

Organism												
Klebsiella spp.												
K. oxytoca	+	+	0	0	0	+	0	+	+	+	0^+	+
K. pneumoniae	+	+	0	0	0	+	0	+	+	+	0^+	0
Morganella morganii	0	+	+^0	v	0	v	+	+	0	0	+^0	+
Proteus spp.												
P. mirabilis	0	+	+	+	0	0	+	+	v	v	+	0
P. vulgaris	0	+	+	0	0	0	+	+	0^+	0	+	+
Providencia spp.												
P. rettgeri	0	+	+	0	0	0	+	+	+	0	+	+
P. stuartii	0	+	+^0	0	0	0	+	v	+	0	+	+
Salmonella spp.	0	+	+	+	+^0	+	0	0	+	0	+	0
Serratia spp.												
S. liquefaciens	0^+	+	+	+^0	0	+^0	0	0	+	+^0	+^0	0
S. marcescens	0	+	+^0	+	0	+	0	0^+	v	+	0^+	0
Shigella sonnei	0	+	0	+	0	0	0	0	0	0	+	0
Yersinia spp.												
Y. enterocolitica	0	+	0	+	0	0	0	v	0	0	+^0	v
Y. pestis	0	+	0	0	0	0	0	0	0	0	0	0

Microbial Identification

Table 5.24 Differential characteristics of selected species of *Vibrio*, *Aeromonas*, and *Plesiomonas*

Species	Growth in NaCl				Arginine dihydrolase	Lysine decarboxylase	Ornithine decarboxylase	Esculin hydrolysis	Voges-Proskauer	Citrate	Acid from:					
	None	1%	8%	10%							Arabinose	Mannitol	Sucrose	Salicin	Cellobiose	Lactose
V. cholerae	+	+	0	0	0	+	+	0	V	+	0	+	+	0	0	0
V. parahaemolyticus	0	+	+^{0}	0	0	+	+	0	0	0	V	+	0	0	0	0
V. alginolyticus	0	+	+	V	0	+	V	0	+	0	0	+	+	0	0	0
V. vulnificus	0	+	0	0	0	+	V	V	0	V	0	V	0^{+}	+	+	+^{0}
V. damsela	0	+	0	0	+	V	0	0	+	0	0	0	0	0	0	0
V. fluvialis	0	+	V	0	+	0	0	0	0	+	+	+	+	0	V	0
A. hydrophila	+	+	0	0	+	+	0	+	+	V	V	+	+	+	0	0
A. caviae	+	+	0	0	+	0	0	+	0	V	+	+	+	+	(+)	+
A. veronii biovar sobria	+	+	0	0	+	+	0	0	+	0	0	+	+	0	V	0
P. shigelloides	+	+	0	0	+	+	+	V	0	0	0	0	0	V	0	0

Table 5.25 Differential characteristics of selected species of *Campylobacter*, *Arcobacter*, and *Helicobacter*

Species	Catalase	Nitrate reductase	H$_2$S on TSI[a]	Hydrolysis Hippurate	Hydrolysis Indoxyl acetate	Growth at 15°C	Growth at 25°C	Growth at 42°C	Growth in 3.5% NaCl	Growth in 1% glycine	Nalidixic acid	Cephalothin
C. coli	+	+	0	0	+	0	0	+	0	+	S	R
C. fetus subsp. *fetus*	+	+	0	0	0	0	+	0	0	+	V	S
C. hyointestinalis	+	+	+	0	0	0	+	+	0	+	R	S
C. jejuni subsp. *jejuni*	+	+	0	+	+	0	0	+	0	+	S	R
C. lari	+	+	0	0	0	0	0	+	0	+	R	R
C. sputorum biovar bubulus	0	+	+	0	0	0	0	+	+	+	R	S
C. sputorum biovar sputorum	0	+	+	0	0	0	0	+	0	+	S	S
C. upsaliensis	W	+	0	0	+	0	0	+	0	V	S	S
A. butzleri	W	+	0	0	+	+	+	V	V	+	S	R
A. cryaerophilus group 1B	+	V	0	0	+	+	+	0	0	0	S	V
H. pylori	+	0	0	0	0	0	0	0	0	0	R	S
H. cinaedi	+	+	0	0	0	0	0	0	0	+	S	V
H. fennelliae	+	0	0	0	+	0	0	0	0	+	S	S

[a] TSI, triple sugar iron.

Microbial Identification

Microbial Identification

Table 5.26 Differential characteristics of selected species of *Pseudomonas* and *Burkholderia*

Species	Oxidase	Growth:			Nitrate reductase	Gelatin hydrolysis	Lysine decarboxylase	Arginine dihydrolase	Acid from:						
		Cetrimide	6.5% NaCl	42°C					Glucose	Fructose	Galactose	Mannose	Xylose	Maltose	Mannitol
P. aeruginosa	+	+°	0	+	V	V	0	+	+	+°	+°	V	+°	0+	V
P. fluorescens	+	+	0	0	0+	+	0	+	+	+	+	+	+	V	+
P. putida	+	+	0	0	0	0	0	+	+	+	+	+	+	0+	0+
P. stutzeri	+	0	+	+°	+	0	0	0	+	+	+	+°	+	+	V
B. cepacia	+	V	NT	V	V	V	+	0	+	+	+	+	+	+	+
B. pseudomallei	+	+	NT	+	+	+	0	+	+	+	+	+	+°	+	+

Table 5.27 Differential characteristics of selected oxidase-negative, nonfermentative, gram-negative bacilli

Species	Motility	Indole	Nitrate reductase	Esculin hydrolysis	Gelatin hydrolysis	Growth at 42°C	Urease	DNase	ONPG[a]	Glucose	Maltose	Sucrose	Mannitol	Xylose
Acinetobacter spp.														
A. baumannii	0	0	0	0	0	+	v	0	0	+	v	0	0	+
A. calcoaceticus	0	0	0	0	0	0	v	0	0	+	v	0	0	0
A. lwoffii	0	0	0	0	0	0	v	0	0	0	v	0	0	0
Chryseomonas luteola (Ve-1)	+	0	v	+	v	v	v	0	+	+	+	0	+	+
Flavimonas oryzihabitans (Ve-2)	+	0	0	0	0	v	v	0	0	+	+	v	+	+
Stenotrophomonas maltophilia	+	0	v	+	+	v	0	+	+	+	+	v	0	v

[a] ONPG, *o*-nitrophenyl-*β*-D-galactopyranoside.

Microbial Identification

Microbial Identification

Table 5.28 Differential characteristics of selected oxidase-positive, nonfermentative, gram-negative bacilli

Species	Indole	Nitrate reductase	Urease	DNase	Esculin	Gelatin	Starch	Polymyxin B	ONPG[a]	Glucose	Maltose	Sucrose	Mannitol	Xylose
					Hydrolysis					Acid from:				
Alcaligenes faecalis	0	0	0	0	0	0	NT	S	0	0	0	0	0	0
Alcaligenes xylosoxidans	0	+	0	0	0	0	NT	S	0	+	0	0	0	+
Agrobacterium radiobacter	0	+	+	0	+	0	NT	S	+	+	+	+	+	+
Ochrobactrum anthropi	0	+	+	0	V	0	NT	S	0	+	V	V	V	+
Sphingomonas paucimobilis	0	0	0	0	+	0	NT	V	+	+	+	+	0	+
Shewanella putrefaciens	0	+	0	+	0	0	0	NT	NT	+	V	V	+	NT
Flavobacterium meningosepticum	+	0	0	+	+	+	0	R	+	+	+	0	+	0
Flavobacterium group IIb	+	V	0	V	+	+	+	R	V	+	+	V	0	V
Weeksella virosa	+	0	0	0	0	+	0	S	0	0	0	0	0	0
Weeksella zoohelcum	+	0	+	0	0	+	0	R	0	0	0	0	0	0

[a] ONPG, *o*-nitrophenyl-β-D-galactopyranoside.

Table 5.29   Catalase and oxidase reactions for selected
gram-negative bacilli

Catalase reaction	Organism	
	Oxidase positive	Oxidase negative or weakly positive
Positive	*Actinobacillus* spp.	*Actinobacillus actinomycetemcomitans*[a]
	Capnocytophaga spp. (DF-2 group)[a]	
	EF-4	
	Pasteurella spp.	
Negative	*Cardiobacterium hominis*[a]	*Capnocytophaga* spp. (DF-1 group)[a]
	Eikenella corrodens[a]	DF-3[a]
	Kingella spp.	
	Suttonella indologenes	

[a] Capnocytophilic.

Microbial Identification

Table 5.30 Differential characteristics of selected catalase-positive, gram-negative bacilli

Species	Oxidase	Nitrate reductase	Indole	Urease	Gelatin	Esculin	Ornithine decarboxylase	Lysine decarboxylase	Arginine dihydrolase	Glucose	Lactose	Maltose	Galactose	Mannitol	Sucrose
Actinobacillus spp.															
A. actinomycetemcomitans	0⁺	+	0	0	0	0	0	0	0	+	0	+	+	+°	0
A. ureae	+	+	0	+	0	0	0	0	0	+	0	+°	0	+	+
Capnocytophaga canimorsus	+	0	0	0	0	V	0	0	+	+	+	+	+°	0	0
EF-4	+	+	0	0	V	0	NT	NT	V	+	0	0	NT	0	0
Pasteurella spp.															
P. canis	+	+	V	0	0	0	+	0	0	+	0	0	+	0	+
P. multocida	+	+	+°	0	0	0	V	0	0	+	0	0⁺	+	+°	+

Table 5.31 Differential characteristics of selected catalase-negative, gram-negative bacilli

Species	Oxidase	Nitrate reductase	Indole	Hydrolysis: Urease	Hydrolysis: Gelatin	Hydrolysis: Esculin	Ornithine decarboxylase	Lysine decarboxylase	Arginine dihydrolase	Acid from: Glucose	Acid from: Lactose	Acid from: Maltose	Acid from: Galactose	Acid from: Mannitol	Acid from: Sucrose
Cardiobacterium hominis	+	0	+	0	0	0	0	0	0	+	0	+	0	+	+
Eikenella corrodens	+	+	0	0	0	0	+	+°	0	0	0	0	NT	0	0
Kingella spp.															
K. denitrificans	+	+	0	0	0	0	NT	NT	NT	+	0	0	0	0	0
K. kingae	+	0	0	0	0	0	NT	NT	NT	+	0	+	0	0	0
Suttonella indologenes	+	0	+	0	0	0	NT	NT	0	+	0	+	NT	0	+
Capnocytophaga spp. (DF-1 group)															
C. gingivalis	0	0	0	0+	0+	V	0	0	0	+	0	+	0	0	+
C. ochracea	0+	0	0	0+	0+	+	0	0	0	+	+	+	+°	0	+
DF-3	0	0	+°	0	0	+	0	0	0	+	+	+	NT	0	+

Microbial Identification

Table 5.32 Differential characteristics of anaerobic, gram-negative bacteria

Species	Kanamycin (1,000 µg)	Vancomycin (5 µg)	Colistin (10 µg)	Growth in 20% bile	Formate or fumate required	Nitrate reductase	Indole	Catalase	Lipase	Urease	Glucose
Bacteroides fragilis group	R	R	R	+	0	0	V	V	0	0	+
Bacteroides ureolyticus	S	R	S	0	+	+	0	0+	0	+	0
Bacteroides gracilis	S	R	S	V	+	+	0	0+	0	0	0
Other *Bacteroides* spp.	R	R	V	0+	0	0	V	0+	0	0	V
Porphyromonas spp.[a]	R	S	R	0	0	0	+	0	0	0	0
Pigmented *Prevotella* spp.[a]	R	R	V	0	0	0	V	0	V	0	+
Other *Prevotella* spp.[a]	R	R	V	0	0	0+	0+	0+	0+	0	+
Bilophila wadsworthia	S	R	S	+	0	+	0	+	0	+0	0
Fusobacterium nucleatum	S	R	S	0	0	0	+	0	0	0	0
Other *Fusobacterium* spp.	S	R	S	V	0	0	+0	0	+0	0	0
Acidaminococcus fermentans	S	R	S	0	0	0	0	0	0	0	0
Megasphaera elsdenii	S	R	S	0	0	0	0	0	0	0	+
Veillonella spp.	S	R	S	0	0	+	0	0+	0	0	0

[a] *Porphyromonas* and some *Prevotella* spp. initially fluoresce red and then develop pigmented colonies.

Table 5.33 Differential characteristics of the *Bacteroides fragilis* group

Bacteroides species	Indole	Catalase	Esculin hydrolysis	α-Fucosidase	Acid from: Arabinose	Cellobiose	Rhamnose	Salicin	Sucrose	Trehalose	Xylan	Metabolic products (GLC)[a]
B. fragilis	0	+	+	+	0	+°	0	0	+	0	0	A, p, S, pa (ib, iv, l)
B. caccae	0	0+	+	+	+	+°	+°	0+	+	+	0	A, p, S (iv)
B. distasonis	0	+°	+	0	0+	+	v	+	+	+	0	A, p, S (pa, ib, iv, l)
B. merdae	0	0+	+	0	0+	v	+	+	+	0	0	A, p, S (ib, iv)
B. vulgatus	0	0+	0+	+	+	0	+	0	+	0	0°	A, p, S
B. thetaiotaomicron	+	+	+	+	+	+°	+°	0+	+	+	0	A, p, S, pa (ib, iv, l)
B. eggerthii	+	0	+	0	+	0+	+°	0	0	0	+	A, p, S (ib, iv, l)
B. ovatus	+	+°	+°	+	+	+	+	+	+	+	+	A, p, S, pa (ib, iv, l)
B. stercoris	+	0	+	v	0+	0+	0+	0+	+	0	v	A, p, S, f (ib, iv)
B. uniformis	+	0+	+	+	+	+	0+	+°	+	0	v	a, p, l, S (ib, iv)

[a] GLC, gas-liquid chromatography.

Mycology

See Flowchart 5.2 and Tables 5.34 and 5.35.

→

Flowchart 5.2 Preliminary identification scheme for yeasts and yeastlike organisms. Growth at ambient temperature but not 37°C: rare *Candida* strains, nonpathogenic *Cryptococcus* spp., and *Geotrichum* spp. Pellicle formation in broth cultures: some *Candida* spp. (not *Candida albicans*) and *Trichosporon, Geotrichum,* and *Blastoschizomyces* spp. Growth on media with cycloheximide: *C. albicans, Candida guilliermondii, Candida kefyr,* and *Blastoschizomyces, Trichosporon,* and *Malassezia* spp.

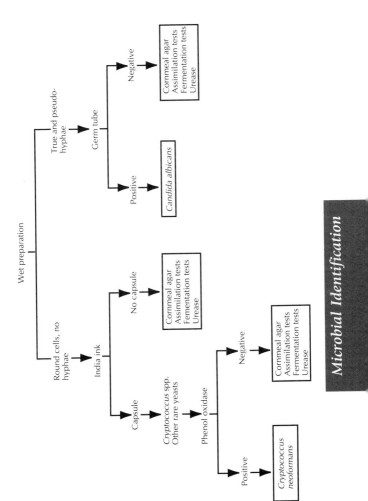

Microbial Identification

Table 5.34 Differential characteristics of fermentative yeasts[a]

Species	Assimilation tests												Fermentation tests						Urease
	Glucose	Maltose	Sucrose	Lactose	Galactose	Melibiose	Cellobiose	Inositol	Xylose	Raffinose	Trehalose	Dulcitol	Glucose	Maltose	Sucrose	Lactose	Galactose	Trehalose	
Candida albicans	+	+	v	0	+	0	0	0	+	0	+	0	+	+	0	0	+	+	0
Candida catenulata	+	+	0	0	+	0	0	0	+	0	0	0	v	0	0	0	0	0	0
Candida guilliermondii	+	+	+	0	+	+	+	0	+	+	0^+	+	+	0	+	0	v	+	0
Candida kefyr	+	0	+	+	+	0	v	0	v	0	0	0	+	0	+	v	+	0	0
Candida krusei	+	0	0	0	0	0	0	0	0	0	0	0	+	0	0	0	0	0	v
Candida lambica	+	0	0	0	0	0	0	0	+	0	0	0	+	0	0	0	0	0	0
Candida lipolytica	+	0	0	0	0	0	0	0	0	0	+	0	0	0	0	0	0	0	+
Candida lusitaniae	+	+	+	0	+	0	+	0	+	0	0	0	+	0	+	0	+	+	0
Candida parapsilosis	+	+	+	0	+	0	0	0	+	0	+	0	+	0	0	0	0	0	0
Candida rugosa	+	0	0	0	+	0	0	0	v	0	+	0	0	+	+	0	0	+	0
Candida tropicalis	+	+	+	0	+	0	0^+	0	+	0	+	0	+	0	0	0	+	0	0
Candida zeylanoides	+	0	0	0	0^+	0	0	0	0	0	+	0	0	0	0	0	0	+	0
Torulopsis glabrata	+	0	0	v	0	+	+	0	0	+	+	v	w	0	w	0	0	w	0
Torulopsis candida	+	+	0	0	+	0	0	0	0	0	0	0	+	0	0	0	0	0	0
Torulopsis pintolopesii	+	+	0	0	0	0	0	0	0	+	v	0	+	0	0	0	0	v	0
Saccharomyces cerevisiae	+	+	+	0	+	0	0	0	0	0	v	0	+	+	+	0	+	+	0
Hansenula anomala	+	+	+	0	+	0	0	0	+	+	+	0	+	+	+	0	+	0	0

[a] The morphology on cornmeal agar must be consistent with the biochemical identification. Strain variations will be observed in individual reactions.

Table 5.35 Identification of nonfermentative yeasts and yeastlike organisms[a]

Species	Assimilation tests												Urease
	Glucose	Maltose	Sucrose	Lactose	Galactose	Melibiose	Cellobiose	Inositol	Xylose	Raffinose	Trehalose	Dulcitol	
Cryptococcus neoformans	+	+	+	0	+	0	+	+	+	>	+	+	+
Cryptococcus albidus	+	+	+	>	>	+	+	+	+	+	+	>	+
Cryptococcus laurentii	+	+	+	+	+	>	+	+	+	>	+	+	+
Cryptococcus luteolus	+	+	+	0	+	0	+	+	+	+	+	+	+
Cryptococcus terreus	+	>	0	>	>	0	+	+	+	0	+	0	+
Cryptococcus uniguttulatus	+	+	+	0	0	0	0	+	+	+	0	0+	+
Rhodotorula glutinis	+	+	+	0	>	0	+	0	+	+	+	0	+
Rhodotorula rubra	+	+	+	0	+	>	>	0	+	+	+	0	0
Trichosporon beigelii	+	+	+	+	>	>	>	+	+	>	>	>	+
Trichosporon pullulans	+	+	+	>	+	0	+	>	>	>	+	0	0
Geotrichum candidum	+	0	0	0	+	0	0	0	+	0	0	0	0
Blastoschizomyces capitatus	+	0	0	0	+	0	0	0	0	0	0	0	0
Prototheca wickerhamii	+	0	0	0	+	0	0	0	0	0	+	0	0

[a] The morphology on cornmeal agar must be consistent with the biochemical identification. Strain variations will be observed in these reactions.

Microbial Identification

Parasitology

See Tables 5.36 to 5.43 and Figures 5.1 to 5.4.

Table 5.36 Trophozoites of common intestinal amebae

Organism	Size[a] (diam or length)	Motility	Nucleus (no. and visibility)	Appearance of stained:			
				Peripheral chromatin	Karyosome	Cytoplasm	Inclusions
Entamoeba histolytica	12–60 μm; usual range, 15–20 μm; invasive forms may be >20 μm	Progressive, with hyaline, fingerlike pseudopodia; may be rapid	1; difficult to see in unstained preparations	Fine granules, uniform in size and usually evenly distributed; may appear beaded	Small, usually compact; centrally located but may also be eccentric	Finely granular, "ground glass"; clear differentiation of ectoplasm and endoplasm; if present, vacuoles are usually small	Noninvasive organism may contain bacteria; erythrocytes, if present, are diagnostic
Entamoeba hartmanni	5–12 μm; usual range, 8–10 μm	Usually nonprogressive	1; usually not seen in unstained preparations	Nucleus may stain more darkly than that of *E. histolytica*, although morphology is similar; chromatin may appear as a solid ring rather than beaded	Usually small and compact; may be centrally located or eccentric	Finely granular	May contain bacteria; no erythrocytes

(continued)

Microbial Identification

Table 5.36 Trophozoites of common intestinal amebae (*continued*)

Organism	Size[a] (diam or length)	Motility	Nucleus (no. and visibility)	Appearance of stained:			
				Peripheral chromatin	Karyosome	Cytoplasm	Inclusions
Entamoeba coli	15–50 μm; usual range, 20–25 μm	Sluggish, nondirectional, with blunt, granular pseudopodia	1; often visible in unstained preparations	May be clumped and unevenly arranged on membrane; may also appear as solid dark ring with no beads or clumps	Large, not compact; may or may not be eccentric; may be diffuse and darkly stained	Granular, with little differentiation into ectoplasm and endoplasm; usually vacuolated	Bacteria, yeast cells, other debris

Endolimax nana	6–12 μm; usual range, 8–10 μm	Sluggish, usually nonprogressive	1; occasionally visible in unstained preparations	Usually no peripheral chromatin; nuclear chromatin may be quite variable	Large irregularly shaped; may appear "blotlike"; many nuclear variations are common; may mimic *E. hartmanni* or *Dientamoeba fragilis*	Granular, vacuolated	Bacteria
Iodamoeba bütschlii	8–20 μm; usual range, 12–15 μm	Sluggish, usually nonprogressive	1; usually not visible in unstained preparations	Usually no peripheral chromatin	Large; may be surrounded by refractile granules that are difficult to see ("basket nucleus")	Coarsely granular; may be highly vacuolated	Bacteria, yeast cells, other debris

[a] Wet-preparation measurements (in permanent stains, organisms usually measure 1 to 2 μm less).
Source: L. S. Garcia and D. A. Bruckner, *Diagnostic Medical Parasitology*, 2nd ed., American Society for Microbiology, Washington, D.C., 1993.

Microbial Identification

Microbial Identification

Table 5.37 Cysts of common intestinal amebae

| Organism | Size[a] (diam or length) | Shape | Nucleus (no. and visibility) | Appearance of stained: | | | |
				Peripheral chromatin	Karyosome	Cytoplasm, chromatoidal bodies	Glycogen[b]
Entamoeba histolytica	10–20 μm; usual range, 12–15 μm	Usually spherical	Mature cyst, 4; immature, 1 or 2; characteristics difficult to see on wet preparation	Fine, uniform granules, evenly distributed; nuclear characteristics may not be as clearly visible as in trophozoite	Small, compact, usually centrally located but occasionally eccentric	May be present; bodies usually elongate with blunt, rounded, smooth edges; may be round or oval	May be diffuse or absent in mature cyst; clumped chromatin mass may be present in early cysts
Entamoeba hartmanni	5–10 μm; usual range, 6–8 μm	Usually spherical	Mature cyst, 4; immature, 1 or 2; 2 nucleated cysts very common	Fine granules evenly distributed on membrane; nuclear characteristics may be difficult to see	Small, compact, usually centrally located	Usually present; bodies usually elongate with blunt, rounded, smooth edges; may be round or oval	May or may not be present, as in *E. histolytica*

Entamoeba coli	10–35 µm; usual range, 15–25 µm	Usually spherical; may be oval, triangular, or other; may be distorted on permanent stained slide owing to inadequate fixative penetration	Mature cyst, 8; occasionally ≥16; immature cysts with ≥2 nuclei occasionally seen	Coarsely granular; may be clumped and unevenly arranged on membrane; nuclear characteristics not as clearly defined as in trophozoite; may resemble *E. histolytica*	Large, may or may not be compact and/or eccentric; occasionally centrally located	May be present (less frequently than in *E. histolytica*); splinter shaped with rough, pointed ends	May be diffuse or absent in mature cyst; clumped mass occasionally seen in mature cysts
Endolimax nana	5–10 µm; usual range, 6–8 µm	Usually oval; may be round	Mature cyst, 4; immature cysts, 2, very rarely seen and may resemble cysts of *Enteromonas hominis*	Rarely present; small granules or inclusions are occasionally seen; fine linear chromatoidal bodies may be faintly visible on well-stained smears	Smaller than karyosome seen in trophozoites but generally larger than those of genus *Entamoeba*	No peripheral chromatin	Usually diffuse if present

Microbial Identification

(continued)

Microbial Identification

Table 5.37 Cysts of common intestinal amebae (*continued*)

Organism	Size[a] (diam or length)	Shape	Nucleus (no. and visibility)	Appearance of stained:			
				Peripheral chromatin	Karyosome	Cytoplasm, chromatoidal bodies	Glycogen[b]
Iodamoeba bütschlii	5–20 μm; usual range, 10–12 μm	May vary from oval to round; cyst may collapse owing to large glycogen vacuole space	Mature cyst, 1	No peripheral chromatin	Larger, usually eccentric refractile granules may be on one side of karyosome ("basket nucleus")	None; small granules are occasionally present	Large, compact, well-defined mass

[a] Wet-preparation measurements (in permanent stains, organisms usually measure 1 to 2 μm less).

[b] Stains reddish brown with iodine.

Source: L. S. Garcia and D. A. Bruckner, *Diagnostic Medical Parasitology*, 2nd ed., American Society for Microbiology, Washington, D.C., 1993.

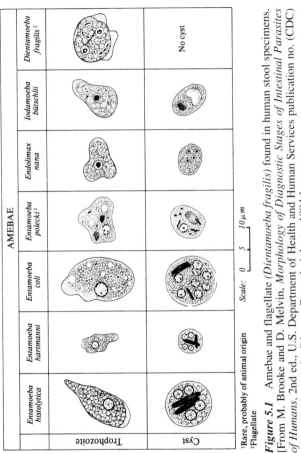

AMEBAE

	Entamoeba histolytica	Entamoeba hartmanni	Entamoeba coli	Entamoeba polecki[1]	Endolimax nana	Iodamoeba bütschlii	Dientamoeba fragilis[2]
Trophozoite							
Cyst							No cyst

[1] Rare, probably of animal origin
[2] Flagellate

Scale: 0   5   10 μm

Figure 5.1 Amebae and flagellate (*Dientamoeba fragilis*) found in human stool specimens. [From M. Brooke and D. Melvin, *Morphology of Diagnostic Stages of Intestinal Parasites of Humans*, 2nd ed., U.S. Department of Health and Human Services publication no. (CDC) 84-8116, Centers for Disease Control, Atlanta, 1984.]

Microbial Identification

Microbial Identification

Table 5.38 Morphologic characteristics of ciliates, coccidia, and tissue protozoa

Species	Shape and size	Other features[a]
Balantidium coli	Trophozoite: ovoid with tapering anterior; 50–100 µm long; 40–70 µm wide (usual width range, 40–50 µm) Cyst: spherical or oval; 50–70 µm in diam (usual range, 50–55 µm)	Trophozoite: 1 large, kidney-shaped macronucleus; 1 small, round micronucleus, which is difficult to see even in stained smears; macronucleus may be visible in unstained preparations; body is covered with cilia, which tend to be longer near cytostome; cytoplasm may be vacuolated Cyst: 1 large macronucleus visible in unstained preparations; micronucleus difficult to see; macronucleus and contractile vacuoles are visible in young cysts; in older cysts, internal structure appears granular; cilia difficult to see within cyst wall
Cryptosporidium parvum	Oocyst generally round, 4–5 µm in diam; each mature oocyst contains sporozoites, which may or may not be visible	Oocyst is the usual diagnostic stage in stool. Various other stages in life cycle can be seen in biopsy specimens taken from GI tract (brush borders of epithelial cells in intestinal tract) and other tissues (respiratory tract, biliary tract).
Cyclospora cayetanensis	Organisms generally round, 8–9 µm in diam; acid-fast like *Cryptosporidium* spp. but larger	Resemble nonrefractile spheres in wet-preparation smears; autofluoresce with epifluorescence; stain variably with acid-fast stains; appear clear, round, and somewhat wrinkled in trichrome stains
Isospora belli	Ellipsoidal oocyst; usual size, 20–30 µm long, 10–19 µm wide; sporocysts rarely seen out of oocysts but measure 9–11 µm	Mature oocyst contains 2 sporocysts with 4 sporozoites each; immature oocysts are usually seen in fecal specimens.

Microsporidia	Spores are extremely small and have been recovered from all body organs.	Histology results vary; acid-fast, trichrome, and calcofluor white stains recommended for spores. Animal inoculation not recommended. Enteric infections in AIDS patients difficult to diagnose by examining stool specimens.
Pneumocystis carinii	Trophozoite: amoeboid shape; about 5 μm long; nucleus visible with Giemsa or hematoxylin stain Cyst: usually round; when mature, contains 8 trophozoites; often 5 μm in diam and contains very small (1-μm) trophozoites	Diagnosis of infections is based on microscopic observation of trophozoites or cysts in clinical (e.g., respiratory) specimens.
Toxoplasma gondii	Trophozoite (tachyzoite): crescent shaped; 4–6 μm long by 2–3 μm wide Cyst (bradyzoite): generally spherical; 200 μm to 1 mm in diam	Diagnosis is most frequently based on clinical history and serologic evidence of infection.
Sarcocystis spp.	Oocyst with thin wall contains 2 mature sporocysts, each containing 4 sporozoites; oocyst frequently ruptures; ovoid sporocysts, each 9–16 μm long and 7.5–12 μm wide	Thin-walled oocyst or ovoid sporocysts occur in stool.

[a] GI, gastrointestinal; PAS, periodic acid-Schiff.

Source: L.S. Garcia and D.A. Bruckner, *Diagnostic Medical Parasitology*. 2nd ed., American Society for Microbiology, Washington, D.C., 1993.

Microbial Identification

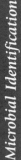

Microbial Identification

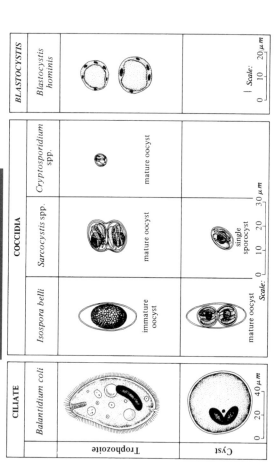

Figure 5.2 Ciliate, coccidia, and *Blastocystis hominis* found in human stool specimens. [From M. Brooke and D. Melvin, *Morphology of Diagnostic Stages of Intestinal Parasites of Humans*, 2nd ed., U.S. Department of Health and Human Services publication no. (CDC) 84-8116, Centers for Disease Control, Atlanta, 1984.]

Table 5.39 Trophozoites of flagellates

Organism	Shape and size	Motility	Nucleus (no. and visibility)	No. of flagella[a]	Other features
Dientamoeba fragilis	Shaped like amebae; 5–15 μm (usual range, 9–12 μm)	Usually nonprogressive; pseudopodia are angular, serrated, or broad lobed and almost transparent	Percentage may vary, but 40% of organisms have 1 nucleus and 60% have 2 nuclei; not visible in unstained preparations; no peripheral chromatin; karyosome is cluster of 4–8 granules	No visible flagella	Cytoplasm finely granular and may be vacuolated with ingested bacteria, yeasts, and other debris; may be great variation in size and shape on single smear
Giardia lamblia	Pear shaped; 10–20 μm long; 5–15 μm wide	Falling-leaf motility may be difficult to see if organism is in mucus	2; not visible in unstained mounts	4 lateral, 2 ventral, 2 caudal	Sucking disk occupying $\frac{1}{2}$–$\frac{3}{4}$ of ventral surface; pear shaped from front, spoon shaped from side

(continued)

Microbial Identification

Microbial Identification

Table 5.39 Trophozoites of flagellates (*continued*)

Organism	Shape and size	Motility	Nucleus (no. and visibility)	No. of flagella[a]	Other features
Chilomastix mesnili	Pear shaped; 6–24 μm long (usual range, 10–15 μm long), 4–8 μm wide	Stiff, rotary	1; not visible in unstained mounts	3 anterior, 1 in cytostome	Prominent cytostome extending ⅓–½ length of body; spiral groove across ventral surface
Trichomonas hominis	Pear shaped; 5–15 μm long (usual range, 7–9 μm long; 7–10 μm wide	Jerky, rapid	1; not visible in unstained mounts	3–5 anterior, 1 posterior	Undulating membrane extends length of body; posterior flagellum extends free beyond end of body
Trichomonas tenax	Pear shaped; 5–12 μm long (usual range, 6.5–7.5 μm), 7–9 μm wide	Jerky, rapid	1; not visible in unstained mounts	4 anterior, 1 posterior	Seen only in preparations from mouth; axostyle (slender rod) protrudes beyond posterior end and may be visible; posterior flagellum extends only halfway down body, and there is no free end

	Shape and size	Motility	Number of nuclei	Number of flagella	Other features
Trichomonas vaginalis	Pear shaped; 7–23 μm long (usual range, 13 μm), 5–15 μm wide	Jerky, rapid	1; not visible in unstained mounts	3–5 anterior; 1 posterior	Undulating membrane extends $\frac{1}{2}$ length of body; no free posterior flagellum; axostyle easily seen
Enteromonas hominis	Oval, 4–10 μm long (usual range, 8–9 μm long), 5–6 μm wide	Jerky	1; not visible in unstained mounts	3 anterior, 1 posterior	One side of body flattened; posterior flagellum extends free posteriorly or laterally
Retortamonas intestinalis	Pear shaped or oval; 4–9 μm long (usual range, 6–7 μm long), 3–4 μm wide	Jerky	1; not visible in unstained mounts	1 anterior, 1 posterior	Prominent cytostome extending approximately $\frac{1}{2}$ length of body

[a] Usually difficult to see.

Source: L.S. Garcia and D.A. Bruckner, *Diagnostic Medical Parasitology*, 2nd ed., American Society for Microbiology, Washington, D.C., 1993.

Microbial Identification

Microbial Identification

Table 5.40 Cysts of flagellates[a]

Species	Size	Shape	Nuclei (no. and visibility)	Other features
Dientamoeba fragilis, Trichomonas hominis, Trichomonas tenax	No cyst stage	NA	NA	NA
Giardia lamblia	8–19 μm long (usual range, 11–14 μm long), 7–10 μm wide	Oval, ellipsoidal, or round	4; not distinct in unstained preparations; usually located at one end	Longitudinal fibers in cysts may be visible in unstained preparations; deeply staining median bodies usually lie across longitudinal fibers; there is often shrinkage, and cytoplasm pulls away from cyst wall; may also be "halo" effect around outside of cyst wall due to shrinkage caused by dehydrating reagents

Chilomastix mesnili	6–10 μm long (usual range, 7–9 μm long), 4–6 μm wide	Lemon shaped with anterior hyaline knob	1; not distinct in unstained preparations	Cytostome with supporting fibrils, usually visible in stained preparation; curved fibril along side of cytostome usually referred to as "shepherd's crook"
Enteromonas hominis	4–10 μm long (usual range, 6–8 μm long), 4–6 μm wide	Elongate or oval	1–4; usually 2 lying at opposite ends of cyst; not visible in unstained mounts	Resembles *Endolimax nana* cyst; fibrils or flagella usually not seen
Retortamonas intestinalis	4–9 μm long (usual range, 4–7 μm long), 5 μm wide	Pear shaped or slightly lemon shaped	1; not visible in unstained mounts	Resembles *Chilomastix* cyst; shadow outline of cytostome with supporting fibrils extends above nucleus; bird beak fibril arrangement

[a] NA, not applicable.

Source: L. S. Garcia and D. A. Bruckner, *Diagnostic Medical Parasitology*, 2nd ed., American Society for Microbiology, Washington, D.C., 1993.

Microbial Identification

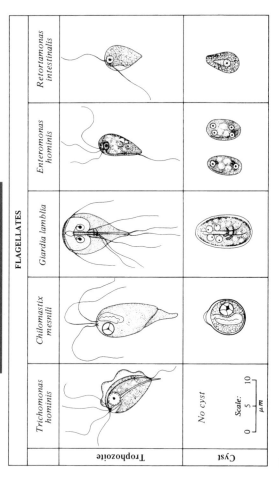

Figure 5.3 Flagellates found in human stool specimens. [From M. Brooke and D. Melvin, *Morphology of Diagnostic Stages of Intestinal Parasites of Humans*, 2nd ed., U.S. Department of Health and Human Services publication no. (CDC) 84-8116, Centers for Disease Control, Atlanta, 1984.]

Table 5.41 Morphologic characteristics of parasites found in blood[a]

Organism	Diagnostic stage
Malaria parasites	
Plasmodium vivax (benign tertian malaria)	Ameboid rings; presence of Schüffner's dots; all stages seen in peripheral blood; mature schizont contains 16–18 merozoites; infects young RBCs
Plasmodium ovale (ovale malaria)	Nonameboid rings; presence of Schüffner's dots; all stages seen in peripheral blood; mature schizont contains 8–10 merozoites; RBCs may be oval and have fimbriated edges; infects young RBCs
Plasmodium malariae (quartan malaria)	Rings are thick; no stippling; all stages seen in peripheral blood; presence of band forms and rosette-shaped mature schizont; lots of malarial pigment; infects mature RBCs
Plasmodium falciparum (malignant tertian malaria)	Multiple rings; appliqué/accolé forms; no stippling (rare Maurer's clefts); rings and crescent-shaped gametocytes seen in peripheral blood (no other developing stages, with rare exception of mature schizont); infects all RBCs
Babesia spp.	Ring forms only (resemble *P. falciparum* rings); seen in splenectomized patients; endemic in the United States (no travel history necessary); if present, "Maltese cross" configuration diagnostic
Trypanosoma brucei gambiense (West African sleeping sickness)	Trypomastigotes long and slender, with typical undulating membrane; lymph nodes and blood can be sampled; microhematocrit tube concentration helpful; examine spinal fluid in later stages of infection

(continued)

Microbial Identification

Microbial Identification

Table 5.41   Morphologic characteristics of parasites found in blood[a] *(continued)*

Organism	Diagnostic stage
Trypanosoma brucei rhodesiense (East African sleeping sickness)	Trypomastigotes long and slender, with typical undulating membrane; lymph nodes and blood can be sampled; microhematocrit tube concentration helpful; examine spinal fluid in later stages of infection
Trypanosoma cruzi (Chagas' disease, South American trypanosomiasis)	Trypomastigotes short and stumpy, often curved in C shape; blood sampled early in infection; trypomastigotes enter striated muscle (heart, GI tract) and transform into amastigote form
Leishmania spp. (cutaneous; not actually a blood parasite but presented for comparison with *Leishmania donovani*)	Amastigotes found in macrophages of skin; presence of intracellular forms containing nucleus and kinetoplast diagnostic
Leishmania braziliensis (mucocutaneous; not actually a blood parasite but presented for comparison with *Leishmania donovani*)	Amastigotes found in macrophages of skin and mucous membranes; presence of intracellular forms containing nucleus and kinetoplast diagnostic
Leishmania donovani (visceral)	Amastigotes found throughout reticuloendothelial system and in spleen, liver, bone marrow, etc.; presence of intracellular forms containing nucleus and kinetoplast diagnostic
Wuchereria bancrofti	Microfilariae sheathed, clear space at end of tail; nocturnal periodicity seen; elephantiasis seen in chronic infections

Brugia malayi	Microfilariae sheathed, subterminal and terminal nuclei at end of tail; nocturnal periodicity seen; elephantiasis seen in chronic infections
Loa loa (African eye worm)	Microfilariae sheathed, nuclei continuous to tip of tail; diurnal periodicity; adult worm may cross conjunctiva of eye
Mansonella spp.	Microfilariae unsheathed, nuclei may or may not extend to tip of tail (depending on species); nonperiodic; symptoms usually absent or mild
Mansonella streptocerca	Microfilariae unsheathed, nuclei extend to tip of tail; when immobile, curved like shepherd's crook; adults in dermal tissues
Onchocerca volvulus	Microfilariae unsheathed, nuclei do not extend to tip of tail; adults in nodules

[a] GI, gastrointestinal; RBCs, erythrocytes.
Source: L. S. Garcia and D. A. Bruckner, *Diagnostic Medical Parasitology,* 2nd ed., American Society for Microbiology, Washington, D.C., 1993.

Microbial Identification

Microbial Identification

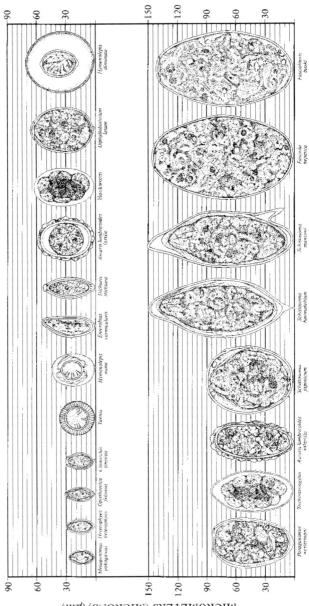

MICROMETERS (MICRONS) (μm)

Figure 5.4 Relative sizes of helminth eggs (from Centers for Disease Control and Prevention). *Schistosoma mekongi* and *Schistosoma intercalatum* have been omitted. [From M. Brooke and D. Melvin, *Morphology of Diagnostic Stages of Intestinal Parasites of Humans,* 2nd ed., U.S. Department of Health and Human Services publication no. (CDC) 84-8116, Centers for Disease Control, Atlanta, 1984.]

Microbial Identification

Table 5.42 Morphologic characteristics of helminths

Helminth	Diagnostic stage
Nematodes (roundworms)	
Ascaris lumbricoides	Egg: both fertilized (oval to round with thick, mammillated or tuberculate shell) and unfertilized (tend to be more oval or elongate, with bumpy shell exaggerated) eggs found in stool. Adult worms: 10–12 in. (ca. 25–30 cm), found in stool. Rarely (in severe infections), migrating larvae can be found in sputum.
Trichuris trichiura	Egg: barrel shaped with two clear, polar plugs. Adult worm: rarely seen. Eggs should be quantitated (rare, few, etc.), since light infections may not be treated.
Enterobius vermicularis	Egg: football shaped with one flattened side. Adult worm: about $\frac{3}{8}$ in. (ca. 1 cm) long, white with pointed tail. Female migrates from anus and deposits eggs on perianal skin.
Ancylostoma duodenale, Necator americanus	Egg: eggs of two species identical; oval with broadly rounded ends, thin shell, and clear space between shell and developing embryo (8–16-cell stage). Adult worms: rarely seen in clinical specimens.
Strongyloides stercoralis	Rhabditiform larvae (noninfective) usually found in stool; short buccal cavity or capsule with large, genital primordial packet of cells (''short and sexy''). In very heavy infections, larvae can occasionally be found in sputum and/or filariform (infective) larvae can be found in stool (slit in tail).
Ancylostoma braziliensis	Humans are accidental hosts. Larvae will wander through outer layer of skin, creating tracks (severe itching and eosinophilia). There are no practical microbiological diagnostic tests.

Toxocara cati or *Toxocara canis*

Humans are accidental hosts. Dog or cat ascarid eggs are ingested with contaminated soil; larvae wander through deep tissues (including eye); can be mistaken for cancer of eye; serologic tests helpful for confirmation; eosinophilia

Cestodes (tapeworms)

Taenia saginata

Scolex (4 suckers, no hooklets) and gravid proglottid (>12 branches on single side) are diagnostic; eggs indicate *Taenia* spp. only (thick, striated shell, containing 6-hooked embryo or oncosphere); worm usually approx 12 ft (ca. 3.7 m) long

Taenia solium

Scolex (4 suckers with hooklets) and gravid proglottid (<12 branches on single side) are diagnostic; eggs indicate *Taenia* spp. only (thick, striated shell, containing 6-hooked embryo or oncosphere); worm usually approx 12 ft (ca. 3.7 m) long

Diphyllobothrium latum

Scolex (lateral sucking grooves) and gravid proglottid (wider than long, reproductive structures in center, "rosette"); eggs operculated

Hymenolepis nana

Adult worm not normally seen; egg round to oval with thin shell, containing 6-hooked embryo or oncosphere with polar filaments lying between embryo and egg shell

Hymenolepis diminuta

Adult worm not normally seen; egg round to oval with thin shell, containing 6-hooked embryo or oncosphere with no polar filaments lying between embryo and egg shell

Echinococcus granulosus

Adult worm found only in carnivores (dog); hydatid cysts develop (primarily in liver) when humans accidentally ingest eggs from dog tapeworms; cyst contains daughter cysts and many scolices. Laboratory should examine fluid aspirated from cyst at surgery.

(continued)

Microbial Identification

Microbial Identification

Table 5.42 Morphologic characteristics of helminths *(continued)*

Helminth	Diagnostic stage
Echinococcus multilocularis	Adult worm found only in carnivores (fox or wolf); hydatid cysts develop (primarily in liver) when humans accidentally ingest eggs from carnivore tapeworms. Cyst grows like metastatic cancer with no limiting membrane.
Trematodes (flukes)	
Fasciolopsis buski	Eggs found in stool; very large and operculated (morphology like that of *Fasciola hepatica* eggs)
Fasciola hepatica	Eggs found in stool; cannot be differentiated from those of *F. buski*
Clonorchis (Opisthorchis) sinensis	Eggs found in stool; very small (<35 μm); operculated, with shoulders into which operculum fits
Paragonimus westermani	Eggs coughed up in sputum (brownish "iron filings" = egg packets); can be recovered in sputum or stool (if swallowed); eggs operculated, with shoulders into which operculum fits
Schistosoma mansoni	Eggs recovered in stool (large lateral spine); specimens should be collected with no preservatives (to maintain egg viability); worms in veins of large intestine
Schistosoma haematobium	Eggs recovered in urine (large terminal spine); specimens should be collected with no preservatives (to maintain egg viability): worms in veins of bladder
Schistosoma japonicum	Eggs recovered in stool (very small lateral spine); specimens should be collected with no preservatives (to maintain egg viability): worms in veins of small intestine

Source: L. S. Garcia and D. A. Bruckner, *Diagnostic Medical Parasitology*, 2nd ed., American Society for Microbiology, Washington, D.C., 1993.

Table 5.43 Key to adult stages of common arthropods of medical importance

---

1. Three or four pairs of legs [2]
   Five or more pairs of legs [22]

2. Three pairs of legs with antennae **(insects: class Insecta)** [3]
   Four pairs of legs without antennae **(spiders, ticks, mites, scorpions: class Arachnida)** [20]

3. Wings present, well developed [4]
   Wings absent or rudimentary [12]

4. One pair of wings **(flies, mosquitos, midges: order Diptera)** [5]
   Two pairs of wings [6]

5. Wings with scales **(mosquitos: order Diptera)**
   Wings without scales **(other flies: order Diptera)**

6. Mouthparts adapted for sucking, with elongate proboscis [7]
   Mouthparts adapted for chewing, without elongate proboscis [8]

7. Wings densely covered with scales, proboscis coiled **(butterflies and moths: order Lepidoptera)**
   Wings not covered with scales; proboscis not coiled but directed backward **(bedbugs and kissing bugs: Hemiptera)**

8. Both pairs of wings membranous, with similar structure, although size may vary [9]
   Front pair of wings leathery or shell-like, serving as covers for second pair [10]

9. Two pairs of wings similar in size **(termites: order Isoptera)**
   Hind wing much smaller than front wing **(wasps, hornets, and bees: order Hymenoptera)**

10. Front wings horny or leathery without distinct veins, meeting in a straight line down the middle [11]
    Front wings leathery or paperlike with distinct veins, usually overlapping in the middle **(cockroaches: order Dictyoptera)**

11. Abdomen with prominent cerci or forceps; wings shorter than abdomen **(earwigs: order Dermaptera)**
    Abdomen without prominent cerci or forceps; wings covering abdomen **(beetles: order Coleoptera)**

12. Abdomen with three long terminal tails **(silverfish and firebrats: order Thysanura)**
    Abdomen without three long terminal tails [13]

13. Abdomen with narrow waist **(ants: order Hymenoptera)**
    Abdomen without narrow waist [14]

14. Abdomen with prominent pair of cerci or forceps **(earwigs: order Dermaptera)**
    Abdomen without cerci or forceps [15]

15. Body flattened laterally; antennae small, fitting into grooves in side of head **(fleas: order Siphonaptera)**
    Body flattened dorsoventrally; antennae projecting from side of head, not fitting into grooves [16]

(continued)

Table 5.43 Key to adult stages of common arthropods of medical importance *(continued)*

16. Antennae with nine or more segments [17]
    Antennae with three to five segments [18]

17. Pronotum covering head **(cockroaches: order Dictyoptera)**
    Pronotum not covering head **(termites: order Isoptera)**

18. Mouthparts consisting of tubular jointed beak; three- to five-segment tarsi **(bedbugs: order Hemiptera)**
    Mouthparts retracted into head or of chewing type; one- or two-segment tarsi [19]

19. Mouthparts retracted into head, adapted for sucking blood **(sucking lice: order Anopleura)**
    Mouthparts of chewing type **(chewing lice: order Mallophaga)**

20. Body oval, consisting of single saclike region **(ticks and mites: subclass Acari)**
    Body divided into two distinct regions, a cephalothorax and an abdomen [21]

21. Abdomen joined to cephalothorax by slender waist; abdomen with segmentaiton indistinct or absent; stinger absent **(spiders: subclass Araneae)**
    Abdomen broadly joined to cephalothorax; abdomen distinctly segmented, ending with stinger **(scorpions: subclass Scorpiones)**

22. Five to nine pairs of legs or swimmerets; one or two pairs of antennae; principally aquatic organisms **(copepods, crabs, and crayfish: class Crustacea)**
    Ten or more pairs of legs; swimmerets absent; one pair of antennae; terrestrial organisms [23]

23. Only one pair of legs per body segment **(centipedes: class Chilopoda)**
    Two pairs of legs per body segment **(millipedes: class Diplopoda)**

Sources: J. Goddard, *Physician's Guide to Arthropods of Medical Importance,* CRC Press, Inc., Boca Raton, Fla, 1993, and National Communicable Disease Center, *Pictorial Keys: Arthropods, Reptiles, Birds, and Mammals of Public Health Significance,* Communicable Disease Center, Atlanta, 1969.

Microbial Identification

Antimicrobial Agents and Susceptibility Testing

The antimicrobial susceptibility results for an individual isolate form the basis of specific, directed therapy. Additionally, the known susceptibility patterns for groups of organisms are used to guide empiric therapy. Reviewing all the testing methods that are currently available or the results of the numerous studies that have determined susceptibility patterns for all bacteria, fungi, viruses, and parasites would be impossible. For detailed information about the specifics of susceptibility tests, refer to the relevant documents from the National Committee for Clinical Laboratory Standards (see Table 6.1), *Manual of Clinical Microbiology*, 6th ed. (1995), and *Clinical Microbiology Procedures Handbook* (1992). Information on susceptibility patterns is summarized in a number of texts on infectious disease, including *Principles and Practice of Infectious Diseases*, 4th ed. (1995), *Antibiotics in Laboratory Medicine*, 3rd ed. (1991), and *The Use of Antibiotics*, 4th ed. (1989). The material presented here is divided into three parts and presented in tabular form. The first part (Tables 6.1, 6.2, and 6.3) summarizes antimicrobial susceptibility testing information. The second part (Tables 6.4 and 6.5) lists common antibiotics used to treat bacterial, fungal, viral, and parasitic infections and summarizes general pharmacokinetic values for these drugs. The last part (Tables 6.6 through 6.14) summarizes the spectra of activity of various antimicrobial agents. Material presented in this section was derived from the books listed above and from other relevant published literature.

Antimicrobial Agents

Table 6.1 National Committee for Clinical Laboratory Standards documents relevant to antimicrobial susceptibility testing

No.[a]	Title
M2-A5	Performance Standards for Antimicrobial Disk Susceptibility Tests (1993)
M6-T	Protocols for Evaluating Dehydrated Mueller-Hinton Agar (1993)
M7-A3	Methods for Dilution Antimicrobial Susceptibility Tests for Bacteria That Grow Aerobically (1993)
M11-A3	Methods for Antimicrobial Susceptibility Testing of Anaerobic Bacteria (1993)
M21-T	Methodology for the Serum Bactericidal Test (1992)
M23-A	Development of In Vitro Susceptibility Testing Criteria and Quality Control Parameters (1994)
M24-T	Antimycobacterial Susceptibility Testing for *Mycobacterium tuberculosis* (1995)
M26-T	Methods for Determining Bactericidal Activity of Antimicrobial Agents (1992)
M27-T	Reference Method for Broth Dilution Antifungal Susceptibility Testing of Yeasts (1995)
M33	Antiviral Susceptibility Testing (under development)
M100-S6	Performance Standards for Antimicrobial Susceptibility Testing (1995)

[a] A, approved; M, microbiology standard; P, pending; S, supplement; T, tentative.

Antimicrobial Agents

Antimicrobial Agents

Table 6.2 Summary of antibiotic susceptibility test methods for bacteria, mycobacteria, and fungi

Organism	Test method	Medium[a]	Incubation conditions
Staphylococcus spp.	Disk diffusion	MHA	24 h, air
	Broth microdilution	CAMHB	24 h, air
	Agar dilution	MHA + 2% NaCl	24 h, air
	Agar screen	MHA + 4% NaCl + oxacillin (6 μg/ml)	24 h, air
Streptococcus pneumoniae	Disk diffusion	MHA-B	20–24 h, 5% CO_2
	Broth microdilution	CAMHB + 2–5% LHB	20–24 h, air
Other *Streptococcus* spp.	Disk diffusion	MHA-B	18–24 h, air or CO_2
	Broth microdilution	CAMHB + 2–5% LHB	18–24 h, air or CO_2
	Agar dilution	MHA-B or MHA with LHB	18–24 h, air or CO_2
Enterococcus spp.	Disk diffusion	MHA	16–18 h (24 h, VAN), air
	Broth microdilution	CAMHB	16–18 h (24 h, VAN), air
	Agar screen	BHIA + GEN (500 μg/ml)	24–48 h, air
		BHIA + STR (2,000 μg/ml)	24–48 h, air
		BHIA + VAN (6 μg/ml)	24 h, air

	Method	Medium	Incubation
	Broth screen	BHIB + GEN (500 μg/ml)	24–48 h, air
	Broth screen	BHIB + STR (1,000 μg/ml)	24–48 h, air
Listeria spp.	Disk diffusion	MHA-B	18–24 h, air
	Broth microdilution	CAMHB + 2–5% LHB	18 h, air
Neisseria gonorrhoeae	Disk diffusion	GCA + 1% supplement	20–24 h, 5–7% CO_2
	Agar dilution	GCA + 1% supplement	20–24 h, 5–7% CO_2
Neisseria meningitidis	Disk diffusion	MHA	18–24 h, 5–7% CO_2
	Broth microdilution	CAMHB	24 h, 5–7% CO_2
	Agar dilution	MHA	24 h, 5–7% CO_2
Moraxella catarrhalis	Disk diffusion	MHA	18–24 h, air
	Broth microdilution	CAMHB	18–24 h, air
Haemophilus spp.	Disk diffusion	HTM	16–18 h, 5–7% CO_2
	Broth microdilution	HTM; CAMHB + supplement	20–24 h, air
Family *Enterobacteriaceae*	Disk diffusion	MHA	16–18 h, air
	Broth microdilution	CAMHB	16–18 h, air

(continued)

Antimicrobial Agents

Antimicrobial Agents

Table 6.2 Summary of antibiotic susceptibility test methods for bacteria, mycobacteria, and fungi *(continued)*

Organism	Test method	Medium[a]	Incubation conditions
Pseudomonas spp.	Disk diffusion	MHA	16–18 h, air
	Broth microdilution	CAMHB	16–18 h, air
Acinetobacter spp.	Disk diffusion	MHA	16–18 h, air
	Broth microdilution	CAMHB	16–18 h, air
Anaerobes	Broth microdilution	Various broths	48 h, anaerobic
	Agar dilution	WCB; brucella broth	48 h, anaerobic
Nocardia spp.	Broth microdilution	CAMHB	2–5 days at 35°C, air
Mycobacteria, rapid growers	Broth microdilution	CAMHB + 0.02% Tween 80	3–5 days at 30°C, air
	Agar disk elution	MHA + OADC	3–5 days at 30°C, air
Mycobacteria, slow growers	Proportion agar dilution	7H10 agar + OADC	3 wk at 37°C, 5–10% CO_2
	Radiometric (BACTEC) broth	BACTEC 12B broth	5–14 days at 37°C, BACTEC
Fungi and yeasts	Broth microdilution	RPMI 1640 broth	2–3 days at 35°C, air

[a] Abbreviations: BHIA, brain heart infusion agar; BHIB, brain heart infusion broth; CAMHB, cation-adjusted Mueller-Hinton broth; CAMHB + LHB, CAMHB supplemented with lysed horse blood; GCA, gonococcal agar; GEN, gentamicin; HTM, *Haemophilus* test medium; LHB, lysed horse blood; MHA, Mueller-Hinton agar; MHA-B, MHA supplemented with 5% sheep blood; OADC, oleic acid supplement; STR, streptomycin; VAN, vancomycin; WCB, Wilkins-Chalgren broth.

Table 6.3 Quality control organisms for antimicrobial susceptibility tests

Quality control organism	Test(s)
Staphylococcus aureus ATCC 25923	Disk diffusion
Staphylococcus aureus ATCC 29213	Broth dilution
Enterococcus faecalis ATCC 29212	Disk diffusion and broth dilution
Escherichia coli ATCC 25922	Disk diffusion and broth dilution
Escherichia coli ATCC 35218	Disk diffusion and broth dilution
Pseudomonas aeruginosa ATCC 27853	Disk diffusion and broth dilution
Haemophilus influenzae ATCC 49247	Disk diffusion and broth dilution
Haemophilus influenzae ATCC 49766	Disk diffusion and broth dilution
Neisseria gonorrhoeae ATCC 49226	Disk diffusion and broth dilution
Streptococcus pneumoniae ATCC 49619	Disk diffusion and broth dilution
Bacteroides fragilis ATCC 25285	Agar and broth dilution
Bacteroides thetaiotaomicron ATCC 29741	Agar and broth dilution
Eubacterium lentum ATCC 43055	Agar and broth dilution
Nocardia asteroides ATCC 19247	Broth dilution
Mycobacterium tuberculosis ATCC 27294	Agar dilution and BACTEC
Mycobacterium fortuitum ATCC 6841	Agar elution and broth dilution
Candida albicans ATCC 90028	Broth dilution
Candida albicans ATCC 90029	Broth dilution
Candida parapsilosis ATCC 90018	Broth dilution
Torulopsis glabrata ATCC 90030	Broth dilution
Cryptococcus neoformans ATCC 90112	Broth dilution
Cryptococcus neoformans ATCC 90113	Broth dilution

Antimicrobial Agents

Antimicrobial Agents

Table 6.4 Common antibiotics: generic and trade names

Generic name	Trade name(s)	Trade name	Generic name
Acyclovir	Zovirax	Achromycin	Tetracycline
Albendazole	Zentel	Aerosporin	Polymyxin B
Amantadine	Symmetrel	Albamycin	Novobiocin
Amikacin	Amikin	Alferon	Interferon
p-Aminosalicylic acid	Paser	Amikin	Amikacin
Amoxicillin	Amoxil	Amoxil	Amoxicillin
Amoxicillin-clavulanate	Augmentin	Ancef	Cefazolin
Amphotericin B	Fungizone	Ancobon	Flucytosine
Ampicillin	Omnipen, Polycillin	Anspor	Cephradine
Ampicillin-sulbactam	Unasyn	Aralen	Chloroquine
Azithromycin	Zithromax	Atabrine	Quinacrine
Aztreonam	Azactam	Augmentin	Amoxicillin-clavulanate
Capreomycin	Capastat	Azactam	Aztreonam
Carbenicillin	Geocillin, Geopen	AZT	Zidovudine
Cefaclor	Ceclor	Bactocill	Oxacillin
Cefadroxil	Duricef	Bactrim	Trimethoprim-sulfamethoxazole
Cefamandole	Mandol	Biaxin	Clarithromycin
Cefazolin	Ancef, Kefzol	Bicillin	Penicillin G
Cefixime	Suprax	Biltricide	Praziquantel

Cefmetazole	Zefazone	Capastat	Capreomycin
Cefonicid	Monocid	Ceclor	Cefaclor
Cefoperazone	Cefobid	Cefadyl	Cephapirin
Ceforanide	Precef	Cefizox	Ceftizoxime
Cefotaxime	Claforan	Cefobid	Cefoperazone
Cefotetan	Cefotan	Cefotan	Cefotetan
Cefoxitin	Mefoxin	Ceftin	Cefuroxime
Cefpodoxime	Vantin	Cefzil	Cefprozil
Cefprozil	Cefzil	Celbenin	Methicillin
Ceftazidime	Fortaz, Tazicef, Tazidime	Chloromycetin	Chloramphenicol
Ceftizoxime	Cefizox	Cinobac	Cinoxacin
Ceftriaxone	Rocephin	Cipro	Ciprofloxacin
Cefuroxime	Ceftin, Zinacef	Claforan	Cefotaxime
Cephalexin	Keflex	Cleocin	Clindamycin
Cephalothin	Keflin	Coly-Mycin M	Colistin
Cephapirin	Cefadyl	Cytovene	Ganciclovir
Cephradine	Anspor, Velosef	Daraprim	Pyrimethamine
Chloramphenicol	Chloromycetin	ddC	Zalcitabine
Chloroquine	Aralen	ddI	Didanosine
Cinoxacin	Cinobac	Dendrid	Idoxuridine

(continued)

Antimicrobial Agents

Antimicrobial Agents

Table 6.4 Common antibiotics: generic and trade names *(continued)*

Generic name	Trade name(s)	Trade name	Generic name
Ciprofloxacin	Cipro	Diflucan	Fluconazole
Clarithromycin	Biaxin	Doryx	Doxycycline
Clindamycin	Cleocin	Duracillin	Penicillin G
Clofazimine	Lamprene	Duricef	Cefadroxil
Clotrimazole	Lotrimin, Mycelex	Dynapen	Dicloxacillin
Cloxacillin	Tegopen	Ecostatin	Econazole
Colistin	Coly-Mycin M	Erythrocin	Erythromycin
Cycloserine	Seromycin	Famvir	Famciclovir
Dicloxacillin	Dynapen	Fansidar	Sulfadoxine-pyrimethamine
Didanosine	ddI, Videx	Flagyl	Metronidazole
Diethylcarbamazine	Hetrazan	Floxin	Ofloxacin
Doxycycline	Doryx, Vibramycin	Flumadin	Rimantadine
Econazole	Ecostatin	Fortaz	Ceftazidime
Enoxacin	Penetrex	Foscavir	Foscarnet
Erythromycin	Erythrocin, Pediamycin	Fulvicin	Griseofulvin
Erythromycin-sulfisoxazole	Pediazole	Fungizone	Amphotericin B
Ethambutol	Myambutol	Furoxone	Furazolidone
Ethionamide	Trecator	Gantrisin	Sulfisoxazole
Famciclovir	Famvir	Garamycin	Gentamicin

Fluconazole	Diflucan	Geocillin	Carbenicillin
Flucytosine	Ancobon	Geopen	Carbenicillin
Foscarnet	Foscavir	Gramicidin	Polymyxin B
Furazolidone	Furoxone	Grifulvin	Griseofulvin
Ganciclovir	Cytovene	Grisactin	Griseofulvin
Gentamicin	Garamycin	Hetrazan	Diethylcarbamazine
Griseofulvin	Fulvicin, Grifulvin, Grisactin	Hivid	Zalcitabine
Idoxuridine	Dendrid, Stoxil	Kantrex	Kanamycin
Imipenem	Primaxin	Keflex	Cephalexin
Interferon	Alferon	Keflin	Cephalothin
Iodoquinol	Yodoxin	Kefzol	Cefazolin
Isoniazid	Nydrazid	Lamprene	Clofazimine
Itraconazole	Sporanox	Lariam	Mefloquine
Kanamycin	Kantrex	Lorabid	Loracarbef
Ketoconazole	Nizoral	Lotrimin	Clotrimazole
Lomefloxacin	Maxaquin	Macrobid	Nitrofurantoin
Loracarbef	Lorabid	Macrodantin	Nitrofurantoin
Mebendazole	Vermox	Mandol	Cefamandole
Mefloquine	Lariam	Maxaquin	Lomefloxacin

(continued)

Antimicrobial Agents

Antimicrobial Agents

Table 6.4 Common antibiotics: generic and trade names *(continued)*

Generic name	Trade name(s)	Trade name	Generic name
Mepacrine	Quinacrine	Mefoxin	Cefoxitin
Meropenem	Merrem	Merrem	Meropenem
Methicillin	Celbenin, Staphcillin	Mezlin	Mezlocillin
Metronidazole	Flagyl, Prostostat	Minocin	Minocycline
Mezlocillin	Mezlin	Mintezol	Thiabendazole
Miconazole	Monistat	Monistat	Miconazole
Minocycline	Minocin	Monocid	Cefonicid
Nafcillin	Nafcil, Unipen	Myambutol	Ethambutol
Nalidixic acid	NegGram	Mycelex	Clotrimazole
Neomycin	Mycifradin	Mycifradin	Neomycin
Netilmicin	Netromycin	Mycostatin	Nystatin
Niclosamide	Niclocide	Nafcil	Nafcillin
Nitrofurantoin	Macrobid, Macrodantin	Nebcin	Tobramycin
Norfloxacin	Noroxin	NegGram	Nalidixic acid
Novobiocin	Albamycin	Netromycin	Netilmicin
Nystatin	Mycostatin	Niclocide	Niclosamide
Ofloxacin	Floxin	Nizoral	Ketoconazole
Oxacillin	Bactocill, Prostaphlin	Noroxin	Norfloxacin
Pefloxacin	Peflacine	Nydrazid	Isoniazid

Generic name	Trade name	Generic name	Trade name
Penicillin G	Bicillin, Duracillin	Ampicillin	Omnipen
Penicillin V	Pen-Vee K	p-Aminosalicylic acid	Paser
Pentamidine	Pentam	Erythromycin	Pediamycin
Piperacillin	Pipracil	Erythromycin-sulfisoxazole	Pediazole
Piperacillin-tazobactam	Zosyn	Pefloxacin	Peflacine
Polymyxin B	Aerosporin, Gramicidin	Enoxacin	Penetrex
Praziquantel	Biltricide	Pentamidine	Pentam
Pyrimethamine	Daraprim	Penicillin V	Pen-Vee K
Quinacrine	Atabrine	Piperacillin	Pipracil
Ribavirin	Virazole	Ampicillin	Polycillin
Rifampin	Rifadin, Rimactane	Ceforanide	Precef
Rimantadine	Flumadin	Imipenem	Primaxin
Spectinomycin	Trobicin	Trimethoprim	Proloprim
Stavudine	Zerit	Oxacillin	Prostaphlin
Sulfadoxine-pyrimethamine	Fansidar	Metronidazole	Prostostat
Sulfisoxazole	Gantrisin	Mepacrine	Quinacrine
Tetracycline	Achromycin	Zidovudine	Retrovir
Thiabendazole	Mintezol	Rifampin	Rifadin
Ticarcillin	Ticar	Rifampin	Rimactane
Ticarcillin-clavulanate	Timentin	Ceftriaxone	Rocephin

(continued)

Antimicrobial Agents

Antimicrobial Agents

Table 6.4 Common antibiotics: generic and trade names *(continued)*

Generic name	Trade name(s)	Trade name	Generic name
Tobramycin	Nebcin	Septra	Trimethoprim-sulfamethoxazole
Trimethoprim	Proloprim, Trimpex	Seromycin	Cycloserine
Trimethoprim-sulfamethoxazole	Bactrim, Septra	Sporanox	Itraconazole
Vancomycin	Vancocin	Staphcillin	Methicillin
Zalcitabine	ddC, Hivid	Stoxil	Idoxuridine
Zidovudine	AZT, Retrovir	Suprax	Cefixime
		Symmetrel	Amantadine
		Tazicef	Ceftazidime
		Tazidime	Ceftazidime
		Tegopen	Cloxacillin
		Ticar	Ticarcillin
		Timentin	Ticarcillin-clavulanate
		Trecator	Ethionamide
		Trimpex	Trimethoprim
		Trobicin	Spectinomycin

Unasyn	Ampicillin-sulbactam
Unipen	Nafcillin
Vancocin	Vancomycin
Vantin	Cefpodoxime
Velosef	Cephradine
Vermox	Mebendazole
Vibramycin	Doxycycline
Videx	Didanosine
Virazole	Ribavirin
Yodoxin	Iodoquinol
Zefazone	Cefmetazole
Zentel	Albendazole
Zerit	Stavudine
Zinacef	Cefuroxime
Zithromax	Azithromycin
Zosyn	Piperacillin-tazobactam
Zovirax	Acyclovir

Antimicrobial Agents

Antimicrobial Agents

Table 6.5 Pharmacokinetic properties of antibacterial, antifungal, antiviral, and antiparasitic agents

Antimicrobial agent	Unit dose	Avg peak level in serum (μg/ml) after dose given:		
		p.o.	i.m.	i.v.
Abendazole	15 mg/kg	0.8		
Acyclovir	200 mg	0.6		
	5 mg/kg			8.8
Amantadine	200 mg	0.2–0.9		
Amikacin	7.5 mg/kg		15–20	20–40
p-Aminosalicylic acid	4 g	7–8		
Amoxicillin	500 mg	6–8		
Amoxicillin-clavulanate	500/125 mg	4.4 (AMX)		
		2.3 (CLV)		
Amphotericin B	0.65 mg/kg	1.8–3.5		
Ampicillin	500 mg	2.5–5	8–10	
Ampicillin-sulbactam	1 g			40
	3 g		18 (AMP)	120 (AMP)
			13 (SUL)	60 (SUL)
	1.5 g			
Azithromycin	500 mg	0.4		

Aztreonam	1 g		45	90–160
Capreomycin	1 g		30–35	
Carbenicillin	1 g		20–30	150
Carbenicillin indanyl sodium	764 mg	10		
Cefaclor	500 mg	16		
Cefadroxil	500 mg	10		
Cefamandole	1 g		20–36	90–140
Cefazolin	1 g		65	185
Cefepime	1 g		30	65
Cefixime	400 mg	3.5		
Cefmetazole	1 g			70
Cefonicid	1 g		98	220
Cefoperazone	1 g		65–75	153
Ceforanide	1 g		70	125
Cefotaxime	1 g		20	40–45
Cefotetan	1 g		50–80	160
Cefoxitin	1 g		20–25	55–110
Cefpirome	1 g			86
Cefpodoxime	200 mg	2.3	45	
Cefprozil	500 mg	10.5		

(continued)

Antimicrobial Agents

Antimicrobial Agents

Table 6.5 Pharmacokinetic properties of antibacterial, antifungal, antiviral, and antiparasitic agents *(continued)*

Antimicrobial agent	Unit dose	Avg peak level in serum (μg/ml) after dose given:		
		p.o.	i.m.	i.v.
Ceftazidime	1 g		40	70
Ceftizoxime	1 g		39	80–90
Ceftriaxone	500 mg		40–45	
	1 g			150
Cefuroxime	750 mg		27	50
Cefuroxime axetil	500 mg	9		
Cephalexin	500 mg	18		
Cephalothin	1 g			30–60
Cephapirin	1 g			40–70
Cephradine	500 mg	16		
	1 g			60–80
Chloramphenicol	1 g	10–18	12	10–15
Cinoxacin	500 mg	15		
Ciprofloxacin	500 mg	2.5		
	400 mg			4.6
Clarithomycin	250 mg	0.5–1		
Clindamycin	300 mg	3	6	
	600 mg			10–12

Clotrimazole	20 mg/kg		0.5–1.5	
Cloxacillin	500 mg		10	
Colistimethate sodium	150 mg	5–6		
Cycloserine	250 mg		10	
Didanosine	300 mg		1.6	
Dirithromycin	500 mg		0.45	
Dicloxacillin	500 mg		15	
Doxycycline	100 mg		2.5	4
Enoxacin	400 mg		3–5	
Erythromycin	500 mg		2–3	
	1 g			10
Ethambutol	25 mg/kg		5	
Ethionamide	250 mg		2	
Famciclor	500 mg		3–4	
Fleroxacin	400 mg		5	7–8
Fluconazole	400 mg/kg		4.1–8.0	
5-Flucytosine	2 g		45	50
Foscarnet	57 mg/kg			575 µmol/liter
Fusidic acid	500 mg		25–30	50
Ganciclor	5 mg/kg			8.3

Antimicrobial Agents

(continued)

Antimicrobial Agents

Table 6.5 Pharmacokinetic properties of antibacterial, antifungal, antiviral, and antiparasitic agents *(continued)*

Antimicrobial agent	Unit dose	Avg peak level in serum (μg/ml) after dose given:		
		p.o.	i.m.	i.v.
Gentamicin	1.5 mg/kg		4–6	4–8
Griseofulvin	1 g	1–2		
Imipenem	500 mg			25–35
Isoniazid	300 mg	7		
	800 mg	10–15		
Itraconazole	200 mg	1.1–2.3		
Kanamycin	7.5 mg/kg		20–25	
Ketoconazole	200 mg	3–4.5		
	400 mg	7		
Lomefloxacin	400 mg	3		
Loracarbef	400 mg	14		
Mefloquine	250 mg	0.3		
	1 g	0.5–1.2		
Meropenem	500 mg			25–35
Metronidazole	500 mg	12		20–25
Mezlocillin	1 g		15	
	3 g			260

Miconazole	200 mg	0.1		1.6
Minocycline	1 g	0.5–1		
	100 mg	1		
Nafcillin	500 mg		5–8	20–40
	1 g			
Nalidixic acid	1 g	20–50		
Netilmicin	2 mg/kg		5–7	6–8
Nitrofurantoin	100 mg	<2		
Norfloxacin	400 mg	1.5		
Ofloxacin	400 mg	4		
Oxacillin	500 mg	4–6	14–16	
	1 g			40
Oxytetracycline	250 mg	3–4		
Pefloxacin	400 mg	3		
Penicillin G	500 mg	1.5–2.5		
Aqueous	1×10^6 U		8–10	10
Benzathine	1.2×10^6 U		0.1–0.15	
Procaine	1.2×10^6 U		3	
Penicillin V	500 mg	3–5		
Pentamidine	4 mg/kg			0.5–3.4

(continued)

Antimicrobial Agents

Antimicrobial Agents

Table 6.5 Pharmacokinetic properties of antibacterial, antifungal, antiviral, and antiparasitic agents *(continued)*

Antimicrobial agent	Unit dose	Avg peak level in serum (μg/ml) after dose given:		
		p.o.	i.m.	i.v.
Piperacillin	2 g		36	
	4 g			240
Piperacillin-tazobactam	2.25 g		38 (PIP)	
			7 (TAZ)	
	4.5 g			280 (PIP)
				35 (TAZ)
Polymyxin B	2.5 mg/kg			5
Pyrazinamide	0.5 g	5		
	3 g	30		
Pyrimethamine	25 mg	0.1–0.3		
Quinine	650 mg	3–10		
Ribavirin	1 g	1–3		
Rifampin	600 mg	7–9		10
Rimantadine	200 mg	0.4		
Spectinomycin	2 g			100
Spiramycin	2 g	3		
Stavudine	70 mg	1.4		
Streptomycin	1 g		25–50	

Antimicrobial agent	Dose			
Sulfadiazine	2 g		100–150	
Sulfadoxine	1 g		50–75	
Sulfamethizole	2 g		60	
Sulfamethoxazole	1 g		40	
Sulfisoxazole	2 g		170	
Teicoplanin	200 mg	7		20–40
	400 mg			8
Tetracycline	500 mg		4	
Ticarcillin	1 g	20–30		190
	3 g			
Ticarcillin-clavulanate	3.1 g			330 (TIC); 8 (CLV)
Tobramycin	1.5 mg/kg	4–6		4–8
Trimethoprim	100 mg		1	
Trimethoprim-sulfamethoxazole	160/800 mg		3 (TMP); 46 (SMX)	9 (TMP); 106 (SMX)
Vancomycin	500 mg			20–40
Zalcitabine	0.5 mg		7.6 ng/ml	
Zidovudine	200 mg		1.1	

[a] Abbreviations: p.o., perorally; i.m., intramuscularly; i.v., intravenously; AMP, ampicillin; PIP, piperacillin; SMX, sulfamethoxazole; SUL, sulbactam; TAZ, tazobactam; TIC, ticarcillin; CLV, clavulanate; TMP, trimethoprim.

Source: Adapted from P. R. Murray, E. J. Baron, M. A. Pfaller, F. C. Tenover, and R. H. Yolken, *Manual of Clinical Microbiology,* 6th ed., p. 1300, American Society for Microbiology, Washington, D.C., 1995, and A. Kucers and N. M. Bennet, *The Use of Antibiotics,* 4th ed., J. B. Lippincott Co., Philadelphia, 1989.

Antimicrobial Agents

Abbreviations and Footnotes for Tables 6.6 through 6.11

S, isolates generally susceptible; R, isolates generally resistant; V, isolates with variable susceptibility pattern; NA, data not available.

Aminoglycoside group: gentamicin, tobramycin, amikacin, and netilmicin; Beta-lactam combination: ampicillin-sulbactam and amoxicillin-clavulanate; Ceph, 1st, narrow-spectrum cephalosporins; Ceph, 2nd, expanded-spectrum cephalosporins and cephamycins; Ceph, 3rd, broad-spectrum cephalosporins; Erythromycin group: erythromycin and azithromycin; Penicillin group: carbenicillin, mezlocillin, and piperacillin; Quinolone group: ciprofloxacin and ofloxacin; Tetracycline group: tetracycline, doxycycline, and minocycline; TMP-SMX, trimethoprim-sulfamethoxazole.

Table 6.6 Spectra of activity of antibacterial agents against common gram-positive bacteria

Bacteria	Ampicillin	Beta-lactam combination	Penicillin	Oxacillin	Ceph, 1st	Chloramphenicol	Clindamycin	Erythromycin	Gentamicin	Tetracycline group	TMP-SMX	Vancomycin
Staphylococcus aureus (1)	S	S	S	S	S	S	S	S	S	S	S	S
Staphylococcus aureus (2)	R	S	R	S	S	S	S	S	S	V	S	S
Staphylococcus aureus (3)	R	S	R	S	S	S	R	R	S	V	S	S
Staphylococcus aureus (4)	R	R	R	R	R	V	R	R	V	V	V	S
Staphylococcus aureus (5)	R	S	R	R	R	S	S	S	S	S	S	S
Staphylococcus aureus (6)	R	R	R	R	R	S	S	S	S	S	S	S
Staphylococcus spp., coagulase negative	V	V	V	V	V	V	V	V	V	V	V	S
Group D, *Enterococcus* spp.	V	V	V	R	R	S	R	V	R	R	R	V
Group D, nonenterococci	S	S	S	S	S	S	S	S	R	S	S	S
Streptococcus pneumoniae and other streptococci	V	V	V	S	S	S	S	S	R	S	S	S
Listeria monocytogenes	S	S	S	S	R	S	S	S	S	S	S	S

Antimicrobial Agents

Antimicrobial Agents

Table 6.7 Spectra of activity of antibacterial agents against miscellaneous gram-positive bacteria

Bacterial genus or species	Ampicillin	Beta-lactam combination	Penicillin	Oxacillin	Ceph, 1st	Chloramphenicol	Clindamycin	Erythromycin	Gentamicin	Tetracycline group	TMP-SMX	Vancomycin	Quinolone group
Aerococcus	NA	NA	V	R	S	NA	S	R	R	S	R	S	R
Bacillus anthracis	NA	NA	S	NA	S	NA	S	S	S	S	NA	NA	NA
Bacillus cereus	R	R	R	NA	NA	S	S	S	S	S	S	R	S
Erysipelothrix	S	S	S	NA	S	V	S	V	R	V	R	R	S
Lactobacillus	V	NA	S	NA	S	NA	S	NA	NA	NA	NA	R	NA
Leuconostoc	V	V	V	NA	R	S	NA	S	S	NA	S	R	NA
Nocardia	R	V	R	NA	NA	NA	NA	R	V	V	S	NA	R
Oerskovia	S	S	S	NA	NA	NA	NA	R	V	R	S	S	R
Pediococcus	V	V	V	NA	R	S	NA	NA	S	NA	S	R	NA
Rhodococcus	R	S	R	R	R	V	S	S	S	S	V	S	S
Stomatococcus	V	S	S	S	S	S	S	S	R	V	V	S	S

Table 6.8 Spectra of activity of antibacterial agents against common members of the family *Enterobacteriaceae*

Bacterial genus or species	Ampicillin	Beta-lactam combination	Penicillin group	Ceph, 1st	Ceph, 2nd	Ceph, 3rd	Imipenem	Aminoglycoside group	Quinolone group	TMP-SMX	Tetracycline group	Chloramphenicol	Erythromycin group
Citrobacter (diversus) koseri	R	V	V	S	S	S	S	S	S	S	S	S	R
Citrobacter freundii	R	V	V	R	V	V	S	S	S	V	S	S	R
Enterobacter aerogenes	R	V	V	R	V	V	S	S	S	S	S	S	R
Enterobacter cloacae	R	V	V	R	V	V	S	S	S	S	S	S	R
Enterobacter agglomerans	V	S	S	V	V	S	S	S	S	S	S	S	R
Escherichia coli (1)	S	V	S	S	S	S	S	S	S	S	S	S	R
Escherichia coli (2)	R	V	V	V	S	S	S	S	S	S	V	V	R
Klebsiella	R	V	V	V	S	S	S	S	S	S	S	S	R
Morganella	R	V	S	R	S	S	S	S	S	S	V	S	R
Proteus mirabilis	V	V	S	S	V	S	S	S	S	S	R	S	R
Proteus vulgaris	R	V	S	R	R	S	S	S	S	S	R	S	R
Providencia	R	V	S	R	V	S	S	V	S	S	R	S	R
Salmonella	S	S	S	S	S	V	S	S	S	S	S	S	R
Serratia	R	R	S	R	R	S	S	S	S	S	R	S	R
Shigella	S	S	S	S	S	S	S	S	S	V	S	S	R

Antimicrobial Agents

Antimicrobial Agents

Table 6.9 Spectra of activity of antibacterial agents against other gram-negative bacilli

Bacterial genus or species	Ampicillin	Beta-lactam combination	Penicillin group	Ceph, 1st	Ceph, 2nd	Ceph, 3rd	Imipenem	Aminoglycoside group	Quinolone group	TMP-SMX	Tetracycline group	Chloramphenicol	Erythromycin
Acinetobacter anitratus	R	V	S	R	R	S	S	S	S	S	V	R	R
Actinobacillus	V	V	S	V	V	S	S	S	S	S	S	S	V
Aeromonas	R	V	V	R	R	S	S	S	S	S	V	S	R
Bartonella	V	V	V	V	V	V	NA	NA	V	V	S	S	S
Bordetella pertussis	V	S	S	R	R	S	NA	NA	S	V	V	S	S
Borrelia	S	S	S	R	R	S	R	R	S	R	S	S	S
Brucella	R	R	R	R	R	V	NA	S	S	V	S	S	R
Burkholderia cepacia	R	R	V	R	R	V	R	R	R	S	R	S	R
Campylobacter coli	V	S	V	R	R	S	S	S	S	V	S	S	R

Organism													
Campylobacter jejuni	V	S	V	S	S	R	R	V	S	S	S	S	V
Capnocytophaga	V	S	V	V	S	V	V	S	S	S	S	S	V
Cardiobacterium	S	R	S	S	S	S	S	S	S	S	NA	S	V
Chromobacterium	R	R	S	R	S	R	R	V	S	S	S	S	R
Eikenella	S	S	S	S	NA	S	R	S	NA	R	S	NA	NA
Francisella	R	R	V	R	S	R	S	S	S	S	S	V	S
Haemophilus influenzae	V	S	V	S	S	S	S	S	V	V	S	V	V
Helicobacter pylori	S	S	S	S	S	S	S	S	S	V	S	NA	S
Kingella	S	S	S	S	S	S	S	S	S	R	S	S	S
Leptospira	S	S	S	S	S	S	R	NA	NA	NA	NA	R	NA
Legionella	V	S	V	V	V	R	V	NA	NA	NA	NA	NA	S
Pasteurella	S	S	S	S	S	S	R	S	S	S	S	S	R
Plesiomonas	R	R	R	S	R	R	R	S	S	S	S	R	R
Pseudomonas aeruginosa	R	R	R	R	V	R	R	V	R	S	R	R	R
Pseudomonas stutzeri	V	V	V	V	S	R	V	V	R	S	V	R	R
Stenotrophomonas maltophilia	R	R	R	S	V	R	R	R	R	R	R	S	R
Streptobacillus	S	S	S	S	S	S	S	NA	NA	S	S	S	S
Vibrio	V	S	S	NA	NA	NA	NA	S	NA	S	NA	NA	S

Antimicrobial Agents

Table 6.10 Spectra of activity of antibacterial agents against cell wall-defective and intracellular bacteria

Bacterial genus or species	Ampicillin	Beta-lactam combination	Penicillin	Oxacillin	Ceph, 1st	Chloramphenicol	Clindamycin	Erythromycin	Gentamicin	Tetracycline group	TMP-SMX	Vancomycin	Quinolone group
Chlamydia	R	R	R	R	R	NA	S	S	NA	S	S	R	S
Coxiella	R	R	R	R	R	V	R	R	R	S	S	R	S
Ehrlichia	R	R	R	R	R	R	R	R	R	S	R	R	R
Mycoplasma pneumoniae	R	R	R	R	R	V	S	S	V	S	R	R	V
Rickettsia	R	R	R	R	R	S	R	S	R	S	R	R	S
Ureaplasma	R	R	R	R	R	V	R	S	V	S	NA	R	V

Table 6.11 Antimycobacterial agents ranked by clinical utility and expected in vitro susceptibility

	Antimycobacterial agent[b]			
Mycobacterium species[a]	Primary or first choice	Secondary or second choice	Alternative or investigational	Resistance likely
Well documented				
M. tuberculosis, M. africanum, M. bovis[c]	INH, RMP, PZA, STR, EMB	Ciprofloxacin, ofloxacin, ethionamide, cycloserine	Amikacin, rifabutin, sparfloxacin	
M. leprae	Dapsone, RMP, clofazimine	Ethionamide, prothionamide	Clarithromycin, minocycline	
M. avium, M. intracellulare	Azithromycin, clarithromycin, EMB	Amikacin, clofazimine, ciprofloxacin, rifabutin	Cycloserine, STR	INH, PZA
M. chelonae	Amikacin, clarithromycin	Kanamycin		Primary antituberculosis agents, ciprofloxacin, other quinolones

(continued)

Antimicrobial Agents

Antimicrobial Agents

Table 6.11 Antimycobacterial agents ranked by clinical utility and expected in vitro susceptibility *(continued)*

Mycobacterium species[a]	Antimycobacterial agent[b]		
	Primary or first choice	Secondary or second choice	Alternative or investigational	Resistance likely
M. fortuitum	Amikacin, cefoxitin	Cefmetazole, imipenem, minocycline, capreomycin, kanamycin, ciprofloxacin		Primary antituberculosis agents
M. abscessus	Amikacin, clarithromycin	Kanamycin, cefoxitin		Primary antituberculosis agents, ciprofloxacin, other quinolones
Less well documented				
M. kansasii	INH, RMP, EMB	Amikacin, ethionamide, STR, cycloserine		
M. malmoense	INH, RMP, EMB			
M. ulcerans	RMP, amikacin	EMB, TMP-SMX	STR, clofazimine	

M. marinum	RMP, EMB	TMP-SMX, minocycline	Clarithromycin
M. simiae	Insufficient information		
M. haemophilum	Ciprofloxacin, cycloserine, RMP, rifabutin	Azithromycin, clarithromycin, amikacin, clofazimine	Ofloxacin, sparfloxacin
M. scrofulaceum	Excision without chemotherapy?	INH, RMP, STR, cycloserine	
M. szulgai	INH, RMP, EMB	STR, capreomycin, viomycin	
M. xenopi	None	INH, RMP, STR, cycloserine	

[a] For species for which experience is well-documented, primary and secondary agents are listed. For species for which choices are more speculative, largely because of the paucity of available information, first- and second-choice agents are given. First-choice agents are expected to be active against wild-type isolates (i.e., from untreated patients). Second-choice agents are less preferred, usually for reasons of toxicity, expense, or unclear efficacy.

[b] Abbreviations: EMB, ethambutol; INH, isoniazid; PZA, pyrazinamide; RMP, rifampin; STR, streptomycin.

[c] *M. bovis* and *M. bovis* BCG are considered pyrazinamide resistant.

Antimicrobial Agents

Antimicrobial Agents

Table 6.12 Spectra of activity of antifungal agents

Fungus	Amphotericin B	Clotrimazole	Econazole	Fluconazole	5-Flucytosine	Griseofulvin	Itraconazole	Ketoconazole	Miconazole	Nystatin
Yeasts										
Candida	S	S	V	S	V	R	V	S	V	S
Cryptococcus	S	S	V	S	S	R	S	S	S	S
Torulopsis	S	S	V	S	S	R	S	S	S	S
Molds										
Aspergillus	S	S	S	S	R	R	S	V	S	S
Chromoblastomycoses agents	R	S	S	NA	S	R	NA	V	S	NA
Dermatophytes	R	S	S	NA	R	S	S	S	S	S
Entomophthorales	S	R	R	NA	R	R	NA	V	S	NA
Mucorales	S	R	R	NA	R	R	NA	R	R	NA
Mycetoma agents	R	R	S	NA	R	R	NA	V	S	NA
Dimorphic fungi	S	S	S	S	R	R	S	S	V	S

Table 6.13 Antiviral agents generally active against specific viruses

Virus	Antiviral agent(s)
Cytomegalovirus	Foscarnet, ganciclovir, vidarabine
Hepatitis B virus	Foscarnet, interferon
Hepatitis C virus	Interferon
Herpes simplex virus	Acyclovir, foscarnet, ganciclovir, idoxuridine, vidarabine
Human immunodeficiency virus	ddC, ddI, ddT, foscarnet, ribavirin, zidovudine
Influenza A virus	Amantadine, ribavirin, rimantadine
Influenza B virus	Ribavirin
Lassa fever virus	Ribavirin
Papillomavirus	Interferon
Parainfluenza virus	Ribavirin
Respiratory syncytial virus	Ribavirin
Vaccinia virus	Vidarabine
Varicella-zoster virus	Acyclovir, foscarnet, vidarabine

Antimicrobial Agents

Table 6.14 Antiparasitic agents generally active against specific parasites

Parasite	Antiparasitic agent(s)
Protozoa	
Babesia	Clindamycin plus quinine
Balantidium	Tetracycline, iodoquinol, metronidazole
Cyclospora	Trimethoprim-sulfamethoxazole
Dientamoeba	Iodoquinol, tetracycline
Entamoeba	Metronidazole
Giardia	Metronidazole, quinacrine
Isospora	Trimethoprim-sulfamethoxazole
Leishmania	Sodium stibogluconate (CDC[a]), meglumine antimonate, amphotericin B, pentamidine
Naegleria	Amphotericin B
Plasmodium falciparum	
Chloroquine resistant	Quinine plus Fansidar or tetracycline
Chloroquine susceptible	Cloroquine, quinidine
Other *Plasmodium* spp.	Cloroquine or quinidine plus primaquine
Toxoplasma	Fansidar, spiramycin
Trichomonas	Metronidazole
Trypanosoma cruzi	Nifurtimox, benznidazole
Trypanosoma brucei	Suramin (CDC), melarsoprol (CDC), pentamidine
Cestodes	
Cysticercus	Albendazole, praziquantel
Echinococcus	Albendazole
All other tapeworms	Praziquantel, niclosamide
Nematodes	
Dracunculus	Metronidazole, thiabendazole
Enterobius	Pyrantel, mebendazole, albendazole
Filariae	
Onchocerca	Ivermectin (CDC)
All others	Diethylcarbamazine
Strongyloides	Thiabendazole, ivermectin
Toxocara	Diethylcarbamazine, albendazole, mebendazole
Trichostrongylus	Pyrantel pamoate, mebendazole, albendazole
Other nematodes	Mebendazole
Trematodes	
Fasciola	Bithionol (CDC)
All others	Praziquantel

[a] CDC, available through Centers for Disease Control and Prevention.

Immunodiagnostic Tests

Antibody-mediated diagnostic tests are divided into two general categories: tests to detect an organism or its antigenic by-products and structural components (e.g., exotoxins, polysaccharide capsule), and tests to measure the patient's immune response to the infection. Antigen detection tests can be used with a variety of specimens, including blood or serum, cerebrospinal fluid, other normally sterile fluids, urine, and tissue. Antibody detection tests are performed primarily with serum or plasma specimens. The presence of an antigen in a clinical specimen can be interpreted with relative ease, but monitoring a patient's humoral immune response is complex. The presence of antibodies directed against an organism can represent active disease, asymptomatic colonization, or an infection in the recent or distant past. Although high levels or titers of antibodies can be indicative of current infection, most diagnostic procedures require demonstration of a significant increase or decrease in antibodies (e.g., a fourfold or greater change in antibody titer). Interpretation of antibody detection tests is also complicated by the testing method and the patient population under evaluation. For these reasons, general interpretive guidelines are useful but must be supplemented with knowledge of the limitations of the specific test method and other testing variables that influence the requested test.

This chapter consists of three sections: general interpretive guidelines for antibody detection tests, a listing of six reference laboratories that perform specific antibody detection tests and the testing methods they use, and a similar listing for antigen detection tests. The six reference laboratories are among the most commonly used national facilities in the United States. The lists of tests and reference ranges were provided by the test laboratories; however, the selection of tests that each laboratory performs and the testing methods can change. In addition, the laboratories may accept specimens for tests not listed in the tables and refer the specimens to a specialty laboratory for testing. This chapter is a guide to the testing services offered by selected reference laboratories and the interpretation of immunodiagnostic tests. Specific inquiries should be directed to the reference laboratory performing the test. For additional information, please consult the *Manual of Clinical Microbiology,* 6th ed. (1995), or the *Manual of Clinical Laboratory Immunology,* 4th ed. (1992).

Immunodiagnostic Tests

Immunodiagnostic Tests: Interpretive Values

Bacteria

***Bartonella henselae* (Bartonellosis; Cat Scratch Disease).** Immunofluorescence tests appear to be sensitive and specific, with immunoglobulin M (IgM) antibody detected early in the course of disease and IgG antibodies developing later and then declining over time. Approximately 15% of the healthy population have IgG titers of $\geq 1:128$, so a fourfold rise should be demonstrated. Enzyme immunoassays (EIAs) are reported to be equivalent to immunofluorescence tests in sensitivity and specificity.

***Bordetella pertussis* (Pertussis).** Although many different test methods have been evaluated, the enzyme-linked immunoassay appears to be the most promising and popular assay. The test has high sensitivities for detection of antibody rises in paired sera when antibodies to several antigens are measured (e.g., IgG to filamentous hemagglutinin [FHA] and pertussis toxin, IgA to FHA). EIAs for IgA antibodies show promise as rapid diagnostic tests because IgA antibodies are not produced following immunization and are detected only during the acute phase of illness.

***Borrelia* Species (Relapsing Fever).** Many species of relapsing fever spirochetes are not available for preparation of antigens in serologic tests. In addition, spontaneous changes of surface antigens in the spirochetes make serodiagnosis difficult. However, promising results have been obtained with immunofluorescence assays using cultured spirochetes as antigens.

***Borrelia burgdorferi* (Lyme Disease).** Interpretation of serologic tests for Lyme disease is complicated by the observation that significant cross-reactivity has been observed with other species of *Borrelia* and in patients with syphilis, leptospirosis, and periodontal disease. Antibiotic therapy early in the course of disease may also ameliorate antibody responses. Finally, significant variations in commercial reagents and the technological performance of the test contribute to sensitivity and specificity problems. Immunofluorescence tests and EIAs are used extensively, with positive serology confirmed by Western blot (immunoblot) analysis. Efforts to purify species-specific antigens have identified a 39-kDa protein that is conserved among all Lyme disease spirochetes and may resolve the specificity problems with this assay.

Immunodiagnostic Tests

***Brucella* Species (Brucellosis).** A positive agglutination titer is ≥1:80. A fourfold or greater rise in antibody titer indicates active or recent infection. Stable elevated antibody titers are reported in 5 to 10% of the healthy population living in areas of endemic disease, so serology should be used to confirm the clinical diagnosis of brucellosis.

***Chlamydia* Species.** Immunofluorescence tests for infant pneumonitis *(Chlamydia pneumoniae)*, pelvic inflammatory disease *(Chlamydia trachomatis)*, and psittacosis *(Chlamydia psittaci)* have been defined as positive at an IgG antibody titer of ≥1:10. Immunofluorescence tests are the most sensitive assays for chlamydial disease. IgM antibody titers of >1:32 and IgG antibody titers of >1:2,000 are considered diagnostic for lymphogranuloma venereum. Rising antibody titers generally are not demonstrated with this chronic infection. Other infections are diagnosed by a fourfold or greater rise in antibody titer, although this rise may not be observed with chronic or recurrent disease. The immunofluorescence test is genus specific. EIAs do not reliably detect IgM antibody, are less sensitive than the immunofluorescence test for IgG antibody, and are genus specific. The complement fixation antibody test is considered positive at a titer of >1:16. A single antibody titer of >1:64 supports a diagnosis of lymphogranuloma venereum. The test is insensitive for trachoma, inclusion conjunctivitis, or related genital infection and cannot be used to diagnose neonatal infections. It is genus specific.

***Clostridium botulinum* Toxin.** The Centers for Disease Control and Prevention measure the levels of antibodies against *Clostridium botulinum* toxin (antitoxin levels) in patients immunized with toxoid. This test assesses immunity and cannot be used for the diagnosis of botulism. The appropriate diagnostic test for food-borne botulism is a demonstration of botulinal toxin in serum, feces, gastric contents, or vomitus or recovery of the organism from the feces of the patient. Demonstration of the organism or toxin in suspected foods provides indirect evidence of botulism. The presence of the organism or the detection of toxin in wound exudates confirms the diagnosis of wound botulism.

***Clostridium tetani* Toxin.** EIAs have been developed to measure the levels of antibodies against *Clostridium tetani* toxin (antitoxin levels) in patients immunized with toxoid. This test assesses immunity and cannot be used for the diagnosis of tetanus. Levels of $\geq$0.5 IU/ml are generally considered protective. Lower levels indicate that immunization with toxoid may be required. The diagnosis of tetanus is based on clinical parameters; laboratory testing has minimal value.

***Corynebacterium diphtheriae* Toxin.**   EIAs have been developed to measure the levels of antibodies against *C. diphtheriae* toxin (antitoxin levels) in patients immunized with toxoid. These tests assess immunity and cannot be used for the diagnosis of diphtheria. Levels of $\geq$0.01 IU/ml are considered protective. Lower levels indicate that immunization with toxoid may be required. The diagnosis of diphtheria is based on clinical parameters and the recovery of toxin-producing strains of *Corynebacterium diphtheriae* from clinical specimens.

***Coxiella burnetii* (Q Fever).**   Antigenic phase variation occurs with *Coxiella burnetii* infections. In acute self-limited infections, antibodies to the phase II antigen appear first and dominate the immune response. With chronic infections, antibody titers to phase I antigen predominate. The ratio between phase I and phase II responses may be useful for distinguishing between acute and chronic infections. A fourfold or greater increase in antibody titer indicates active or recent infection. A serum titer of $\geq$1:16 in the complement fixation test or $\geq$1:256 in the immunofluorescence test is considered diagnostic.

***Ehrlichia chaffeensis* (Human Monocytic Ehrlichiosis).** The specific etiologic agent for human monocytic ehrlichiosis was isolated in 1990 and is now used to prepare specific antigens for the serologic diagnosis of this disease. Until additional experience is gained with this test, a fourfold or greater increase in IgG antibody titer is considered to indicate active or recent infection. A positive titer for a single serum has not been established. This test will not identify human granulocytic ehrlichiosis, an infection recently attributed to *Ehrlichia equi*.

***Francisella tularensis* (Tularemia).**   A fourfold or greater increase in antibody titer or a single agglutination titer of $\geq$1:160 is considered diagnostic of active or recent infection. Elevated antibody titers late in disease are common, and levels from 1:20 to 1:80 may persist for years. Antibody titers of <1:20 usually represent nonspecific cross-reactions.

Helicobacter pylori.   Gastric disease caused by *H. pylori* is associated with elevated antibody titers. IgM measurement is not clinically useful. Measurement of IgG and IgA antibody titers can be used to diagnose active disease. Elevated antibody levels are present in many adult patients, so diagnosis of active disease is dependent upon detection of a fourfold or greater increase in antibody titer.

Legionella pneumophila **(Legionellosis).** Immunofluorescence antibody titers of ≥1:256 are compatible with current or past infection. A fourfold or greater rise in antibody titer to ≥1:128 indicates active infection. The test sensitivity is approximately 80%. Seroconversion usually occurs within 3 weeks but should be monitored for up to 6 weeks. Some patients fail to produce a diagnostic antibody response. Specificity is greater than 95%, but cross-reactions with a variety of gram-negative and gram-positive bacteria have been observed.

Leptospira **Species (Leptospirosis).** An indirect hemagglutination antibody titer of ≥1:100 is considered to indicate active or recent infection. However, this genus-specific test is considered relatively insensitive. The complement fixation test can be used to determine subgroup specificity, but it, too, lacks sensitivity.

Murine Typhus. Immunofluorescence IgG antibody titers of ≥1:64 are considered to indicate exposure to *Rickettsia typhi*. A fourfold or greater rise in antibody titer indicates active or recent infection.

Mycoplasma pneumoniae. Immunofluorescence IgG and IgM antibody titers of ≥1:10 are considered positive, with active disease indicated by the presence of IgM antibodies or a fourfold or greater rise in IgG antibody titer. The agglutination assay detects IgG and IgM antibodies. A single agglutination antibody titer of ≥1:320 or a fourfold or greater rise in antibody titer indicates active or recent infection. Complement fixation antibody titers of ≥1:64 or a fourfold or greater rise in antibody titer indicates active or recent infection. The specificity of each of these tests is a problem, because cross-reactions with other *Mycoplasma* species have been observed. This problem can be circumvented with the use of the species-specific P1 adhesin protein in the immunoassays.

Rocky Mountain Spotted Fever. Immunofluorescence IgG antibody titers of ≥1:64 are considered to indicate exposure to *Rickettsia rickettsii*. A fourfold or greater rise in titer is consistent with active or recent infection.

Scrub Typhus.   Agglutination antibody titers of $\geq 1:80$ are considered to indicate exposure to *Rickettsia tsutsugamushi*. A fourfold or greater rise in antibody titer indicates active or recent infection.

***Treponema pallidum* (Syphilis).**   Refer to Table 7.1.

Fungi

***Aspergillus* Species.**   The presence of a precipitin band(s) represents a positive immunodiffusion test. A complement fixation antibody titer of $\geq 1:8$ is considered positive. This test is more specific but less sensitive than the immunodiffusion test.

***Blastomyces dermatitidis* (Blastomycosis).**   The presence of precipitin band A indicates a positive immunodiffusion antibody test. A complement fixation antibody titer of $\geq 1:8$ is considered positive. This test is relatively insensitive and nonspecific for blastomycosis. Culture or histology must be used to confirm the serologic results.

***Candida* Species.**   The presence of a precipitin band(s) indicates a positive immunodiffusion assay. The test is nonspecific, because approximately 25% of the healthy population is positive. In addition, the test has poor sensitivity, especially for patients with localized disease.

***Coccidioides immitis* (Coccidioidomycosis).**   Any complement fixation antibody titer with coccidioidin is presumptive evidence for infection. Antibody titers of $1:2$ to $1:4$ usually indicate early, residual, or meningeal disease. Antibody titers of $\geq 1:16$ indicate disseminated disease. Negative titers do not exclude the disease.

***Cryptococcus neoformans* (Cryptococcosis).**   A positive agglutination test suggests infection but does not exclude past exposure or cross-reactions. Negative reactivity during active infection may occur as a result of binding of antibodies by soluble antigen.

***Histoplasma capsulatum* (Histoplasmosis).**   Two specific immunodiffusion bands (H and M) may be present in the sera of patients exposed to *Histoplasma capsulatum*. The M band generally appears first. In the absence of the H band, the M band may be attributed to active disease, inactive disease, or skin test reactivity. The H band is associated with active disease. Two antigens are used in the complement fixation test: yeast and histoplasmin. Complement fixation antibodies to the yeast antigen appear first and reach a higher peak. An antibody titer of ≥1:8 is considered presumptive evidence of disease, although elevated titers are commonly present in healthy patients and in patients with other fungal infections. Antibody titers of ≥1:32 or a fourfold rise in antibody titer is consistent with active or recent infection.

***Penicillium marneffei* (Penicilliosis).** The presence of a precipitin band(s) indicates a positive immunodiffusion assay. No data regarding the sensitivity and specificity of this test are currently available. The test should be used to confirm the clinical diagnosis of penicilliosis. These infections are usually disseminated, with multiple organ involvement such as lymphadenitis, subcutaneous abscesses, bone lesions, arthritis, splenomegaly, or lesions in the lung, liver, or bowel. The diagnostic test of choice is recovery of *P. marneffei* in clinical specimens.

***Sporothrix schenckii* (Sporotrichosis).** Agglutination antibody titers of ≥1:8 are considered positive. A fourfold or greater rise in antibody titer indicates active or recent infection. Antibody titers as high as 1:128 have been reported in patients with localized or disseminated sporotrichosis.

Zygomycetes (Zygomycosis, Mucomycosis). The presence of a precipitin band(s) indicates a positive immunodiffusion assay. This test is rarely used, because the etiologic agents of zygomycosis grow rapidly and are easy to recover in clinical specimens.

Parasites

***Babesia microti* (Babesiosis).** The presence of IgM antibodies is considered a positive agglutination assay. A fourfold or greater increase in IgG antibody is consistent with active or recent infection. Antibody titers rise rapidly during the first weeks of illness and then fall gradually over 6 months to titers of 1:16 to 1:256, remaining at that level for a year or more. Elevated antibody titers are present in healthy individuals who live in areas of endemic infection. Therefore, positive serology should be confirmed with detection of the parasite in blood smears. Cross-reactivity among *Babesia* species is variable, so regional differences in serologic reactivity may be observed.

***Echinococcus* Species (Echinococcosis).** Antibody reactivity in patients infected with *Echinococcus granulosus* is influenced by the location and integrity of the cyst. Antibody response is more common in patients with cysts in bone and liver than in those with cysts in lungs, brain, and spleen. Seroreactivity is always lower in patients with intact cysts. The test sensitivities of indirect hemagglutination assays, indirect fluorescent-antibody assays, and EIA range from 60 to 90%. False-positive reactions may occur in persons with other helminthic infections, cancer, collagen disease, and cirrhosis. Nonspecific reactions have been reduced when purified *Echinococcus multilocularis* antigen was used.

***Entamoeba histolytica* (Amebiasis).** The Centers for Disease Control and Prevention recommend a titer of $\geq 1:256$ as the criterion for positive indirect hemagglutination serology. This level will identify 95% of patients with extraintestinal infections, 70% of patients with active disease localized to the intestines, and 10% of asymptomatic intestinal carriers. Positive titers may persist for 2 years or more. The EIA is a sensitive assay with significantly higher values than the indirect hemagglutination assay in patients with hepatic disease. No cross-reactions with other amebas occur. The immunodiffusion test has been used to confirm positive EIAs but is less sensitive than the indirect hemagglutination assay or EIA. Detection of IgM antibodies is insensitive, even for patients with active invasive disease.

Fasciola hepatica. EIAs using the excretory-secretory antigens are the tests of choice. Specific antibodies appear within 2 to 4 weeks after infection (5 to 7 weeks before eggs appear in stool). Sensitivity approaches 95%; however, cross-reactivity may occur with serum specimens from patients with schistosomiasis. Antibody titers decrease rapidly following treatment, so they can be used to predict the success of therapy.

Filariae (Filariasis). Positive serum antibody tests are of little diagnostic value except in patients not native to areas of filarial endemicity. Most residents of regions where filariae are endemic have high antibody levels. In addition, cross-reactions with other nematode parasites can occur. Serology may be useful for confirming a clinical diagnosis of filariasis in a traveler to an area of endemicity.

***Giardia lamblia* (Giardiasis).** Antibody responses in *Giardia* infections are not commonly monitored, because the antigen can be detected by a variety of immunoassays and microscopy. Greatly elevated antibody titers indicate exposure to the parasite, with a fourfold or greater increase in antibody titer being consistent with active or recent infection.

***Leishmania* spp. (Leishmaniasis).**   The sensitivities of all serologic tests for leishmaniasis are low. Antibody detection may be useful for diagnosing visceral leishmaniasis but is less reliable for cutaneous leishmaniasis, since most patients with this disease fail to produce detectable circulating antibodies. Cross-reactions occur in patients with Chagas' disease.

***Paragonimus westermani* (Paragonimiasis).**   Serologic tests for paragonimiasis include complement fixation, immunofluorescence, EIAs, and immunoblot assays. The tests are highly sensitive and specific. Antibody titers decrease rapidly after successful therapy, so they can be used to monitor response.

***Plasmodium* Species (Malaria).**   Serodiagnosis is recommended for screening blood donors suspected of a previous malarial infection and for testing any patient from an area of endemic disease who has a febrile illness and negative blood smears. The test is sensitive and specific but cannot be used to discriminate between active and past infection. The immunofluorescence test uses antigens from all four *Plasmodium* species associated with human disease.

***Schistosoma* Species (Schistosomiasis).**   Test sensitivity and specificity are highly dependent upon the antigen preparation used and the testing method. EIAs with *Schistosoma mansoni* adult microsomal antigen are sensitive for infections with this species but less so for *Schistosoma japonicum* and *Schistosoma haematobium* infections. Use of immunoblots ensures detection of the other two species if the clinical history suggests these infections. Species specificity is gained in immunoblots when adult worm antigens are used.

***Strongyloides stercoralis* (Strongyloidiasis).**   EIAs are currently recommended as the test of choice, with a sensitivity reported to be between 84 and 92%. Immunocompromised persons typically mount a detectable immune response. Nonreactivity is observed in 8 to 16% of carriers. Cross-reactions can occur in patients with filariasis and some other nematode infections. The highest antibody sensitivity and specificity are obtained when antigens derived from *Strongyloides stercoralis* filariform larvae are used. The tests cannot differentiate between active and and past infection.

Immunodiagnostic Tests

***Taenia solium* (Cysticercosis).** The immunoblot assay has a sensitivity approaching 100% and is more sensitive than other available assays. Seropositivity is reported in 50 to 70% of patients with a single cyst, 80% of patients with multiple calcified lesions, and >90% of patients with multiple non-calcified lesions. EIAs are less sensitive than the immunoblot assay and cross-react with antibodies specific for other helminth infections. Currently available tests do not distinguish between active and inactive infections, so serology cannot be used to evaluate the outcome or prognosis following treatment.

***Toxocara canis* (Visceral-Ocular Larva Migrans).** Antibody tests are the only means of confirming the presumptive diagnosis of toxocaral visceral larva migrans or ocular larva migrans. Larval antigens are used in EIAs. The test sensitivity and specificity cannot be precisely assessed, because alternative methods of demonstrating infection have not been developed. However, the test sensitivity is estimated to vary from 70 to 80% and the specificity is >90%; sensitivity is higher with visceral larva migrans.

***Toxoplasma gondii* (Toxoplasmosis).** The immunofluorescence test is defined as negative when the IgG antibody titer is ≤1:16 (except for ocular infections, in which low titers are commonplace), equivocal at a titer of 1:16 to 1:256, and positive at a titer of >1:256. A positive response is also defined as a fourfold or greater increase in antibody titer. IgM antibody titers of ≥1:64 indicate active infection in adults, and any IgM antibody titer is considered significant in newborns. The sensitivity of the EIA is considered equivalent to that of the immunofluorescence test. Serologic determination of active central nervous system toxoplasmosis in immunocompromised patients is not possible at this time. Specific IgG antibody levels in these patients are often low, and IgM antibodies are generally nondetectable.

***Trichinella spiralis* (Trichinosis).** Detectable antibodies do not develop until 3 to 5 weeks after infection (well after the acute stage of illness), peak in the second or third month, and then decline slowly for several years. Antibodies are detected earlier with the EIA than with other test methods, but the EIA is less specific. Positive EIAs can be confirmed with flocculation tests.

***Trypanosoma cruzi* (Chagas' Disease).** Immunofluorescence can be used to detect IgM and IgG antibody response. The test is very sensitive, but cross-reactivity occurs in patients

Immunodiagnostic Tests

with leishmaniasis, a disease that occurs in the same geographical area. The complement fixation test is less sensitive. An elevated antibody titer cannot be used to differentiate between active and past disease.

Viruses

Adenovirus.   A positive complement fixation antibody titer is $\geq 1:8$. A fourfold or greater rise in titer indicates active or recent infection. The test is relatively insensitive, with only 50 to 70% of patients positive, and the complement fixation test is group specific.

California Encephalitis Virus.   A positive immunofluorescence antibody titer is $\geq 1:8$. A fourfold or greater rise in titer indicates active or recent infection.

Coxsackie A Virus.   A positive complement fixation antibody titer is $\geq 1:8$, although monitoring the patient's antibody response is generally not considered useful. The response is not type specific (nonspecific); may initially be high, making it impossible to demonstrate seroconversion; or can remain negative (insensitive).

Coxsackie B Virus.   A positive complement fixation antibody titer is $\geq 1:8$, although monitoring the patient's antibody response is generally not considered useful. The response is not type specific (nonspecific); may initially be high, making it impossible to demonstrate seroconversion; or can remain negative (insensitive).

Cytomegalovirus.   IgM antibodies measured by EIAs may persist for months to years and can be detectable during reactivated disease. Elevated IgM antibody levels or a fourfold or greater increase in IgG antibodies is consistent with active or recent cytomegalovirus infection. However, the antibody response must be correlated with the clinical status of the patient.

Dengue Virus.   Both IgM and IgG antibodies against all four dengue fever virus types can be detected by the immunofluorescence assay. Cross-reacting IgG antibodies are observed among all four types. In most patients, dengue virus antibodies are detectable after the first week following the onset of symptoms. Cross-reactivity with other arboviruses can occur.

Eastern Equine Encephalitis Virus.   Antibody titers of $\geq 1:8$ are considered positive in the immunofluorescence assay. A fourfold or greater rise in antibody titer indicates active or recent infection.

Echovirus.   Complement fixation antibody titers of $\geq 1:8$ are considered positive. Antibody response is not generally considered useful. The response is not type specific (nonspecific); may initially be high, making it impossible to demonstrate seroconversion; or can remain negative (insensitive).

Epstein-Barr Virus (Infectious Mononucleosis).   Refer to Table 7.2.

Hantavirus.   Hantaviruses are the etiologic agents of hemorrhagic fever with renal syndrome. Antibodies produced by patients with this infection usually cross-react with other viruses in the family. Active or recent infection is suggested by an elevated antibody titer (e.g., $\geq 1:1,024$) or a fourfold or greater increase in titer.

Hepatitis A Virus.   The diagnosis of acute or past infection with hepatitis A virus is assessed by measuring IgM and total antibodies by EIA. IgM antibodies directed against the virus are almost always present in the patient's serum at the time symptoms develop. Total antibody response (IgM, IgG, IgA) develops during the acute phase and persists indefinitely. The presence of IgM alone is consistent with active, acute disease. IgM antibody with a positive total antibody titer is consistent with either active or recent disease, and positive total antibody titer but negative IgM antibody is consistent with a past infection and represents immunity.

Hepatitis B Virus.   Refer to Table 7.3.

HCV.   The diagnosis of hepatitis C virus (HCV) infection is currently achieved by detecting specific antibody by EIA and immunoblot assays that use antigens derived from cloning the HCV genome. If both antibody tests are positive, then there is a high likelihood that the patient is infected.

HDV.   The duration of HBV infection determines the duration of hepatitis D virus (HDV) infection. IgM antibodies directed against HDV are transient in acute infection, and IgG antibodies are often undetectable once the hepatitis B surface antigen disappears, so retrospective serodiagnosis is often difficult.

Herpes Simplex Virus.   The immunofluorescence assay is considered positive when the IgM antibody titer is $\geq 1:10$, while the IgG antibody titer is positive at a titer of $\geq 1:5$. The presence of IgM antibodies or a fourfold rise in IgG antibody titer indicates active or recent infection. Antibody response is not type specific. High antibody levels measured by EIAs are present in the population, and cross-reactions between herpes simplex virus types 1 and 2 occur. These tests are useful only for epidemiologic studies.

Human Herpesvirus 6. The immunofluorescence assay is considered positive when the IgM and IgG antibody titers are $\geq 1:20$. The presence of IgM or a fourfold or greater rise in IgG antibody titer is consistent with active or recent infection.

HIV-1 and HIV-2. EIAs are generally used as highly sensitive and specific screening tests. Most assays use viral antigens obtained from human immunodeficiency virus (HIV)-infected T-lymphocyte cell lines. The preparations are usually rich in p24, p17, gp160, gp120, and gp41 antigens. False-negative reactions can occur when the test is done before seroconversion, when the patient is immunosuppressed, and sometimes when the test is done late in the course of AIDS. Some assays that detect HIV type 1 (HIV-1) cannot detect HIV-2. The Western blot assay is the test most commonly used for confirming the presence of HIV-specific antibodies. Interpretation of the Western blot banding pattern varies depending on the health organization that has established the interpretive criteria.

- Food and Drug Administration: bands for p24 and p31 and for gp41, gp160, or gp120
- Centers for Disease Control and Prevention: any two bands (p24, gp41, or gp160/120)
- American Red Cross: three or more bands with one from *gag, pol,* and *env*

HTLV 1/2. Current serologic procedures (e.g., indirect fluorescent antibody, latex agglutination, EIA) cannot differentiate between human T-cell lymphotropic viruses 1 and 2 (HTLV-1 and HTLV-2). EIA sensitivity is >97%, and specificity is >99%. Despite this, the test parameters are insufficient to permit unequivocal serodiagnosis in a low-prevalence population. Initial reactivity must be confirmed by a test such as immunoblot or the radioimmunoprecipitation assay (RIPA). The criteria established for confirmation of HTLV-1 seropositivity include antibodies against both *env* (gp46 and/or gp61/68) and *gag* (p24) gene products by Western blot or RIPA alone or in combination. A sample is considered indeterminate if antibodies against HTLV-1-specific proteins are detected in combinations other than those just given. Sera with no reactivity to any HTLV-1 proteins are considered negative or false positive. An indeterminate immunoblot is usually followed by a RIPA, which has a higher sensitivity for *env* gp61/68.

Influenza A Virus.   A positive immunofluorescence assay is defined as IgM and IgG antibody titers of $\geq 1:10$. The presence of IgM antibodies or a fourfold rise in IgG antibody titer indicates active or recent infection. The presence of IgG antibodies in the absence of IgM antibodies indicates immunity. An antibody titer of $\geq 1:8$ indicates a positive complement fixation test.

Influenza B Virus.   A positive immunofluorescence assay is defined as IgM and IgG antibody titers of $\geq 1:10$. The presence of IgM antibodies or a fourfold rise in IgG antibody titer indicates active or recent infection. The presence of IgG antibodies in the absence of IgM antibodies indicates immunity. An antibody titer of $\geq 1:8$ indicates a positive complement fixation test.

Lymphocytic Choriomeningitis Virus.   A positive complement fixation antibody titer is $\geq 1:8$. The test is insensitive and is less specific than immunofluorescence tests.

Mumps Virus.   Positive IgM and IgM immunofluorescence antibody titers are $\geq 1:10$ and $\geq 1:5$, respectively. The presence of IgM antibodies or a fourfold rise in IgG antibody titer indicates active or recent infection. The presence of IgG antibodies in the absence of IgM antibodies indicates immunity. The presence of antibodies measured by EIAs is presumptive evidence of immunity except when active disease is suspected.

Parainfluenza Virus.   A positive complement fixation antibody titer is $\geq 1:8$. The test is less sensitive but more specific than hemagglutination inhibition tests or EIA.

Parvovirus B19.   The presence of a band(s) detected by Western blotting indicates active or recent infection. Reactivity for IgG antibodies in EIAs indicates past exposure to virus.

Poliovirus.   A positive complement fixation antibody titer is $\geq 1:8$.

Reovirus.   A positive complement fixation antibody titer is $\geq 1:8$.

Respiratory Syncytial Virus.   A positive immunofluorescence assay is defined as an IgM antibody titer of $\geq 1:10$ or an IgG antibody titer of $\geq 1:10$. The presence of IgM antibodies or a fourfold rise in IgG antibody titer indicates active or recent infection. The presence of IgG in the absence of IgM antibodies indicates immunity. A positive complement fixation antibody titer is $\geq 1:8$.

Rubella Virus. The presence of antibodies measured by EIAs is consistent with past exposure to virus or vaccine and is felt to represent immunity, unless a fourfold or greater rise in antibody titer is observed in a patient with disease compatible with rubella.

Rubeola Virus (Measles). The immunofluorescence assay is defined as positive when the IgM or IgG antibody titers are $\geq 1:10$. The presence of IgM antibodies or a fourfold rise in IgG antibody titer indicates active or recent infection. The presence of IgG antibodies in the absence of IgM antibodies indicates immunity. The presence of antibodies detected by EIAs indicates immunity except when active infection is suspected. Detectable immunity may not persist in vaccinated individuals.

St. Louis Encephalitis Virus. A positive immunofluorescence antibody titer is $\geq 1:10$. A fourfold or greater rise in titer indicates active or recent disease.

Varicella-Zoster Virus. The immunofluorescence assay is defined as positive when the IgM or IgG antibody titers are $\geq 1:10$. The presence of IgM antibodies or a fourfold rise in IgG antibody titer indicates active or recent infection. The presence of IgG antibodies in the absence of IgM antibodies indicates immunity. The presence of antibodies measured by the EIA is consistent with immunity unless the patient has a disease compatible with chickenpox or zoster.

Western Equine Encephalitis Virus. A positive immunofluorescence titer is $\geq 1:10$. A fourfold or greater rise in antibody titer indicates active or recent infection.

Table 7.1   Criteria for diagnosis of syphilis[a]

Early syphilis
  Primary
    Definitive: direct microscopic identification of *T. pallidum* in lesion
    material, lymph node aspirate, or biopsy section
    Presumptive (requires 1 and either 2 or 3)
      1. Typical lesion
      2. Reactive nontreponemal test and no history of syphilis
      3. For persons with history of syphilis, fourfold increase in most
         recent quantitative nontreponemal test titer compared with
         results of past tests
    Suggestive (requires 1 and 2)
      1. Lesion resembling chancre
      2. Sexual contact within preceding 90 days with person who has
         primary, secondary, or early latent syphilis
  Secondary
    Definitive: direct microscopic identification of *T. pallidum* in lesion
    material, lymph node aspirate, or biopsy section
    Presumptive (requires 1 and either 2 or 3)
      1. Skin or mucous membrane lesions typical of secondary
         syphilis
         a. Macular, papular, follicular, papulosquamous, or pustular
         b. Condylomata lata (anogenital region or mouth)
         c. Mucous patches (oropharynx or cervix)
      2. Reactive nontreponemal test titer of $\geq 1:8$ and no previous
         history of syphilis
      3. For persons with history of syphilis, fourfold increase in most
         recent nontreponemal test titer compared with previous test
         results
    Suggestive (requires 1 and 2 and is made only when serologic test
    results are not available)
      1. Presence of clinical manifestations as described above
      2. Sexual exposure within past 6 mo to person with early
         syphilis
  Early latent
    Definitive: Definitive diagnosis does not exist because lesions are
    not present in latent stage.
    Presumptive (requires 1, 2, and 3 or 4)
      1. Absence of signs and symptoms
      2. Reactive nontreponemal and treponemal test results
      3. Nonreactive nontreponemal test within preceding yr
      4. Fourfold increase in nontreponemal test titer compared with
         previous test results for persons with history of syphilis or of
         symptoms compatible with early syphilis
    Suggestive (requires 1 and 2)
      1. Reactive nontreponemal test result
      2. History of sexual exposure within preceding yr

Immunodiagnostic Tests

(continued)

Table 7.1 Criteria for diagnosis of syphilis[a] *(continued)*

Late syphilis

Benign and cardiovascular

Definitive: observation of treponemes in tissue sections by direct microscopic examination with DFAT-TP

Presumptive

1. Reactive treponemal test
2. No known history of treatment for syphilis
3. Characteristic symptoms of benign or cardiovascular syphilis

Neurosyphilis

Definitive (requires 1 and either 2 or 3)

1. Reactive serum treponemal test
2. Reactive VDRL CSF test on spinal fluid sample
3. Identification of *T. pallidum* in CSF or tissue by microscopic examination or animal inoculation

Presumptive (requires 1 and either 2 or 3)

1. Reactive serum treponemal test
2. Clinical signs of neurosyphilis
3. Elevated CSF protein (>40 mg/dl) or leukocyte count (>5 mononuclear cells/ml) in absence of other known causes

Neonatal congenital syphilis

Definitive: demonstration of *T. pallidum* by direct microscopic examination of umbilical cord, placenta, nasal discharge, or skin lesion material

Presumptive (requires 1, 2, and 3)

1. Determination that infant was born to mother who had untreated or inadequately treated syphilis at delivery regardless of findings in infant
2. Infant with reactive treponemal test result
3. One of following additional criteria:
   a. Clinical sign or symptoms of congenital syphilis on physical examination
   b. Abnormal CSF finding without other cause
   c. Reactive VDRL CSF test result
   d. Reactive IgM antibody test specific for syphilis

---

[a] Abbreviations: CSF, cerebrospinal fluid; DFAT-TP, direct fluorescent-antibody test for *T. pallidum* with staining of tissue sections; VDRL, Venereal Disease Research Laboratory.

Source: S. J. Norris and S. A. Larsen, pp. 636–651, *in* P. R. Murray, E. J. Baron, M. A. Pfaller, F. C. Tenover, and R. H. Yolken (ed.), *Manual of Clinical Microbiology,* 6th ed., American Society for Microbiology, Washington, D.C., 1995.

Immunodiagnostic Tests

Table 7.2 Serologic profiles of Epstein-Barr virus-associated syndromes[a]

Antibody-antigen	Nonimmune	Infection			Reactive	BL	NPC
		Current primary	Recent primary	Past			
IgM-VCA	–	+	–	–	–	–	–
IgG-VCA	–	+	+	+	+	++	++
IgA-VCA	–	+ or –	–	–	–	–	++
IgG-EA/D	–	+	+	–	+ or –	–	++
IgA-EA/D	–	–	–	–	Not known	–	++
IgG-EA/R	–	+ or –	+ or –	–	+ or –	++	+ or –
Anti-EBNA	–	–	Low	+	+	+	++

[a] Abbreviations: BL, Burkitt's lymphoma; EA/D, early antigen, diffuse; EA/R, early antigen, restricted; EBNA, Epstein-Barr nuclear antigen; NPC, nasopharyngeal carcinoma; VCA, viral capsid antigen.

[b] –, Negative (<1:10); +, positive (≥1:10).

Source: E. T. Lennette, pp. 905–910, *in* P. R. Murray, E. J. Baron, M. A. Pfaller, F. C. Tenover, and R. H. Yolken (ed.), *Manual of Clinical Microbiology*, 6th ed., American Society for Microbiology, Washington, D.C., 1995.

Immunodiagnostic Tests

Immunodiagnostic Tests

Table 7.3 Interpretation of HBV serologic markers in patients with hepatitis[a]

Assay result[a]			
HBsAg	Anti-HBs	Anti-HBc	Interpretation
Positive	Negative	Negative	Early acute HBV infection. Confirmation is required to exclude nonrepeatable or nonspecific reactivity.
Positive	(±)[b]	Positive	HBV infection, either acute or chronic. Differentiate with IgM anti-HBc. Determine level of infectivity with HBeAg or HBV DNA.
Negative	Positive	Positive	Indicates previous HBV infection and immunity to hepatitis B.
Negative	Negative	Positive	Possibilities include HBV infection in remote past, "low-level" HBV carrier, "window" between disappearance of HBsAg and appearance of anti-HBs, or false-positive reaction. Investigate with IgM anti-HBc and/or challenge with HBsAg vaccine. When present, anti-HBe helps validate anti-HBc reactivity.
Negative	Negative	Negative	Another infectious agent, toxic injury to liver, disorder of immunity, hereditary disease of liver, or disease of biliary tract
Negative	Positive	Negative	Vaccine-type response

[a] Abbreviations: Anti-HBs, antibodies to hepatitis B surface antigen; HBc, antibodies to hepatitis B core antigen; HBe, antibodies to hepatitis e antigen; HBeAg, hepatitis e antigen; HBsAg, hepatitis B surface antigen.

[b] ±, Anti-HBs is usually absent in this situation but may occasionally be present.

Source: F. B. Hollinger and J. L. Dienstag, pp. 1033–1049, *in* P. R. Murray, E. J. Baron, M. A. Pfaller, F. C. Tenover, and R. H. Yoken (ed.), American Society for Microbiology, Washington, D.C., 1995.

Table 7.4 Antibody detection tests for various organisms

Organism	Antibody detection tests[a]					
	Mayo	LCA	BBI-NACL	MRL	SKB	CDC[b]
Bacteria						
Bartonella henselae				IFA		IFA
Bordetella pertussis		IFA	IFA, EIA		IFA	
Borrelia spp. (relapsing fever)			IFA	IFA		EIA
Borrelia burgdorferi (Lyme disease)	EIA, WB	EIA, WB	EIA, WB	IFA, WB	EIA, WB	EIA
Brucella species	AGGL		EIA	IFA	AGGL	AGGL
Chlamydia species	IFA	EIA, IFA	IFA, CF	IFA, CF	EIA, IFA	IFA, CF
Clostridium botulinum toxin						EIA
Clostridium tetani toxin		EIA		EIA	EIA	
Corynebacterium diphtheriae toxin				EIA	EIA	
Coxiella burnetii (Q fever)	IFA	IFA	IFA, CF	IFA	IFA	IFA
Ehrlichia chaffeensis			IFA	IFA		IFA
Escherichia coli O157 toxin						EIA
Francisella tularensis	AGGL	AGGL	AGGL	AGGL	AGGL	

(continued)

Immunodiagnostic Tests

Table 7.4 Antibody detection tests for various organisms *(continued)*

Organism	Antibody detection tests[a]					
	Mayo	LCA	BBI-NACL	MRL	SKB	CDC[b]
Haemophilus influenzae type b						
Helicobacter pylori	EIA	EIA	EIA	EIA	EIA	
Legionella pneumophila	IFA	IFA	IFA, RIA	IFA, RIA	IFA	IFA
Leptospira species	IHA	IHA	IHA	IHA	IHA	IHA
Murine typhus	IFA	IFA			IFA	IFA
Mycoplasma pneumonia	IFA	AGGL	IFA	IFA, EIA, CF	EIA, CF	CF
Rocky Mountain spotted fever	IFA	IFA	IFA		IFA	IFA
Salmonella typhi						IHA
Scrub typhus	AGGL			IFA		IFA
Treponema pallidum	FTA-ABS, RPR, VDRL	FTA-ABS, RPR, MHA-TP, VDRL	FTA-ABS, RPR, VDRL	FTA-ABS, RPR, VDRL	FTA-ABS, RPR, MHA-TP, VDRL	
Yersinia pestis						IHA
Fungi						
Aspergillus species	ID	ID	ID, CIE	ID, CF	ID, CF	ID
Blastomyces dermatitidis	ID	CF	ID, CF	ID, CF	ID, CF	ID, CF, EIA

Candida species	ID	ID	ID	ID			ID, EIA, AGGL
Coccidioides immitis	CF	CF	ID, CF	ID, CF, AGGL	ID, CF	ID, CF	ID, CF
Cryptococcus neoformans		AGGL	IFA	IFA			AGGL
Histoplasma capsulatum	ID	CF	ID, CF	ID, CF			ID, CF
Penicillium marneffei							ID
Sporothrix schenckii	AGGL		AGGL	AGGL			AGGL
Zygomycetes							ID, EIA
Parasites							
Babesia microti	EIA		IFA	IFA			IFA
Echinococcus spp.		IHA	IHA	EIA, WB			IHA, IB
Entamoeba histolytica	IHA	IHA	IHA	EIA, ID	IHA		IHA

(continued)

Immunodiagnostic Tests

Immunodiagnostic Tests

Table 7.4 Antibody detection tests for various organisms *(continued)*

Organism	Antibody detection tests[a]					
	Mayo	LCA	BBI-NACL	MRL	SKB	CDC[b]
Fasciola hepatica				EIA		
Filariasis			IHA			
Giardia lamblia			IFA	EIA		
Leishmania spp.			IFA	IFA		IFA, CF
Paragonimus westermani			IFA	IFA		IB
Plasmodium species			IFA	IFA		IFA
Schistosoma species			EIA	EIA		EIA, IB
Strongyloides stercoralis			EIA	EIA, WB		EIA
Taenia solium (cysticercosis)	EIA		EIA			IB
Toxocara canis	EIA		EIA	EIA		EIA
Toxoplasma gondii	IFA	EIA	EIA	EIA, IFA	EIA	EIA, IFA
Trichinella spiralis (trichinosis)	AGGL		IHA	EIA	EIA	EIA, AGGL
Trypanosoma cruzi (Chagas' disease)			IHA	IFA		IFA, CF
Viruses						
Adenovirus	CF	CF	CF	CF	CF	CF, IHA
California encephalitis virus	IFA	IFA		IFA	IFA	EIA, IHA, CF

Virus						
Colorado tick fever virus				IFA	IFA	EIA, CF
Coronavirus		CF	CF	CF	CF	
Coxsackie A virus		CF	CF	CF	CF	
Coxsackie B virus		EIA	EIA, AGGL	EIA	EIA	EIA
Cytomegalovirus	EIA				EIA	EIA
Dengue virus			IFA	IFA	IFA	EIA, IHA, CF
Eastern equine encephalitis virus		IFA	IFA	IFA	IFA	EIA, IHA, CF
Echovirus		CF	CF	CF	CF	
Epstein-Barr virus						
Early antigen		IFD	IFA	IFA	IFA	
Nuclear antigen		EIA	IFA	IFA	IFA	
Viral capsid antigen		EIA	IFA	IFA	IFA	
Hantavirus		IFA	IFA	IFA		

(continued)

Immunodiagnostic Tests

Immunodiagnostic Tests

Table 7.4 Antibody detection tests for various organisms *(continued)*

Organism	Antibody detection tests[a]					
	Mayo	LCA	BBI-NACL	MRL	SKB	CDC[b]
Hepatitis A virus	EIA	EIA	EIA	EIA	EIA	EIA
Hepatitis B virus						
Core	EIA	EIA	EIA	EIA	EIA	EIA
Surface	EIA	RIA	EIA	EIA	EIA	EIA
e	EIA	EIA	EIA	EIA	EIA	RIA
Hepatitis C virus	EIA, IB	EIA, IB	EIA, IB	EIA	EIA	
Hepatitis D (delta) virus	EIA	EIA	EIA	EIA	EIA	EIA
Herpes simplex virus	IFA	IFA, EIA	IFA, EIA	IFA, EIA, WB	IFA, EIA	EIA
Human herpes virus 6		IFA	IFA	IFA		
Human immunodeficiency virus						
Type 1	EIA, WB	EIA, WB	EIA, WB	EIA, WB	EIA, WB	EIA, WB
Type 2	EIA, WB	EIA, WB	EIA, WB	EIA, WB		EIA, WB
Human T-cell lymphotropic virus 1 and 2	EIA	EIA	EIA, WB	EIA, WB	EIA	EIA, WB
Influenza A virus	IFA	CF	CF	CF	CF	IHA
Influenza B virus	IFA	CF	CF	CF	CF	IHA
Lymphocytic choriomeningitis virus		CF	CF	IFA	CF	IFA
Mumps virus	IFA	EIA, IFA	EIA, IFA	IFA	EIA	IHA

Parvovirus B19	EIA, WB			EIA, WB	EIA, WB		EIA
Parainfluenza virus		CF		CF	CF	CF	IHA
Poliovirus		CF		CF	CF	CF	
Reovirus		CF		CF			
Respiratory syncytial virus	IFA	CF	IFA	CF	CF	CF	EIA
Rubella virus	EIA	EIA	EIA, AGGL	EIA	EIA	EIA	EIA
Rubeola virus	IFA	IFA, EIA		IFA	IFA	EIA	EIA
St. Louis encephalitis virus	IFA	IFA		IFA	IFA	IFA	EIA, IHA, CF
Varicella-zoster virus	IFA	IFA, EIA	IFA, AGGL	IFA, CF	IFA, CF	EIA	IFA
Western equine encephalitis virus	IFA	IFA		IFA	IFA	IFA	EIA, IHA, CF

[a] Abbreviations: Mayo, Mayo Medical Laboratories, Rochester, Minn.; LCA, Laboratory Corportion of America, Burlington, N.C.; BBI-NACL, Boston Biomedica Inc./North American Clinical Laboratories, New Britain, Conn.; MRL, Microbiology Reference Laboratory, Cypress, Calif.; SKB, Smith Kline Beecham, Tucker, Ga.; CDC, Centers for Disease Control and Prevention, Atlanta, Ga.; AGGL, agglutination; CF, complement fixation; EIA, all enzyme-based immunoassay methods; FTA-ABS, fluorescent treponemal antibody (absorbed); IB, immunoblot; ID, immunodiffusion; IFA, all fluorescence-based immunoassay methods; IHA, immune hemagglutination assay; MHA-TP, microhemagglutination assay *(Treponema pallidum)*; RIA, radioimmunoassay; RPR, rapid plasma reagin test; VDRL, venereal disease research laboratory test; WB, Western blot.

[b] The CDC offers an extensive menu of antibody detection tests for viruses in addition to those listed here. These include tests to detect antibodies against the following viruses: Chikungunya virus, Crimean hemorrhagic fever virus, Dengue virus, Hantaan Korean hemorrhagic fever virus, Japanese encephalitis virus, Kyasanur Forest disease virus, La Crosse encephalitis virus, Murray Valley encephalitis virus, Omsk hemorrhagic fever virus, Powassan virus, tick-borne encephalitis virus, Venezuelan equine encephalitis virus, yellow fever virus, Junin virus, Lassa virus, Marburg virus, Ebola virus, Machupo virus, Norwalk virus, vaccinia virus, and rabies virus.

Immunodiagnostic Tests

Immunodiagnostic Tests

Table 7.5 Antigen detection tests for various organisms

Organism	Antigen detection tests used[a]					
	Mayo	LCA	BBI-NACL	MRL	SKB	CDC[b]
Bacteria						
Bacillus anthracis						DFA
Bartonella henselae				PCR		DFA
Bordetella pertussis	DFA, PCR	DFA	DFA	DFA	DFA	
Borrelia spp. (relapsing fever)						DFA
Borrelia burgdorferi (Lyme disease)	PCR	PCR	PCR	PCR		DFA
Brucella species						DFA
Chlamydia trachomatis	DFA, EIA	DFA, PCR	DFA, PCR	DFA, EIA	PROBE	
Clostridium difficile, toxin A		EIA	EIA		EIA	
Clostridium difficile, toxin B	CYTO	CYTO	CYTO	CYTO	CYTO	
Francisella tularensis				DFA		
Haemophilus influenzae	CIE	AGGL	AGGL	AGGL	AGGL	
Legionella species	DFA	DFA, RIA	DFA, RIA	DFA, PROBE	DFA, PROBE	
Mycobacterium tuberculosis		PCR		PCR	PCR	
Neisseria gonorrhoeae	PROBE	PROBE	PROBE		PROBE	
Neisseria meningitidis	CIE	AGGL	AGGL	AGGL	AGGL	

Streptococcus group B	CIE	AGGL	AGGL	AGGL	AGGL	
Streptococcus pneumoniae	CIE	AGGL	AGGL	AGGL	AGGL	
Tropheryma whippelli (Whipple's disease)	PCR					
Yersinia pestis						DFA
Fungi						
Candida species	ID	ID	ID	ID		
Cryptococcus neoformans	AGGL	AGGL	AGGL	AGGL		
Pneumocystis carinii		DFA	DFA			
Parasites						
Cryptosporidium parvum	EIA		DFA	EIA, DFA		
Entamoeba histolytica			EIA	EIA		
Giardia lamblia	EIA	EIA	DFA	EIA	EIA	
Taenia solium (cysticercosis)				PCR		
Toxoplasma gondii				PCR		
Trichinella spiralis				DFA		
Viruses						
Adenovirus	EIA	EIA	EIA	EIA	EIA	EIA
Colorado tick fever virus		PROBE	DFA			IFA
Cytomegalovirus		PCR		PCR		EIA
Epstein-Barr virus				PCR		EIA

(continued)

Immunodiagnostic Tests

Immunodiagnostic Tests

Table 7.5 Antigen detection tests for various organisms (continued)

Organism	Antigen detection tests used[a]					
	Mayo	LCA	BBI-NACL	MRL	SKB	CDC[b]
Hepatitis B virus	PROBE	PCR		PROBE	PROBE, EIA	PROBE
Hepatitis C virus	PCR	PCR	PCR	PCR		
Herpes simplex virus	PCR	PCR	PCR	PCR		IFA, EIA
Human immunodeficiency virus type 1	EIA	EIA, PCR	EIA, PCR	EIA, PCR	EIA, PCR	EIA
Human papillomavirus	PROBE		PROBE		PROBE	
Human T-cell lymphotropic virus 1 and 2		PCR	PCR	PCR		
Influenza A virus		EIA				EIA
JC virus	PCR					
Parainfluenza virus				DFA	DFA	EIA
Parvovirus B19				PROBE		EIA
Respiratory syncytial virus	EIA	EIA		DFA	DFA, EIA	
Rotavirus	EIA	EIA		EIA	EIA, DFA	EIA
Varicella-zoster virus					DFA	

[a] Abbreviations: Mayo, Mayo Medical Laboratories, Rochester, Minn.; LCA, Laboratory Corportion of America, Burlington, N.C.; BBI-NACL, Boston Biomedica Inc./North American Clinical Laboratories, New Britain, Conn.; MRL, Microbiology Reference Laboratory, Cypress, Calif.; SKB, Smith Kline Beecham, Tucker, Ga.; CDC, Centers for Disease Control and Prevention, Atlanta, Ga.; AGGL, agglutination; CIE, counterimmunoelectrophoresis; CYTO, cytotoxicity assay; DFA, direct fluorescent antibody; EIA, all enzyme-based immunoassay methods; ID, immunodiffusion; PCR, polymerase chain reaction; PROBE, nucleic acid probe hybridization; RIA, radioimmunoassay.

[b] The CDC offers an extensive menu of antigen detection tests for viruses in addition to those listed here. These include tests to detect the following viruses: California encephalitis virus, Chikungunya virus, Crimean hemorrhagic fever virus, dengue virus, eastern equine encephalitis virus, Hantaan Korean hemorrhagic fever virus, La Crosse encephalitis virus, Murray Valley encephalitis virus, Omsk hemorrhagic fever virus, Powassan virus, St. Louis encephalitis virus, tick-borne encephalitis virus, Venezuelan equine encephalitis virus, western equine encephalitis virus, yellow fever virus, Junin virus, Lassa virus, Machupo virus, Marburg virus, Ebola virus, Sabia virus, etc. Normally it

Notifiable Infectious Diseases

The epidemiology program at the Centers for Disease Control and Prevention monitors the incidence of selected infectious diseases through state and territorial departments of health. These data are published weekly in *Morbidity and Mortality Weekly Reports* (MMWR), and periodic summaries are published throughout the year. An annual summary report for the preceding year is generally published in October.

The accuracy of the reporting system is dependent on the cooperation of the physicians who see infected patients and the hospital laboratories that confirm the diagnosis. Obviously, physicians and hospitals are the weakest links in the chain, and the reported incidences of some diseases (e.g., gonorrhea, syphilis, salmonellosis) significantly underestimate the true incidences of these diseases in the community. Despite this limitation, important trends can be followed, and the information is instrumental in shaping health care policy.

The list of reportable diseases varies from state to state and year to year, so the data provided in this section should be used as a guideline. Each laboratory has the responsibility to contact its state or local health department to determine which diseases are reportable in its geographic area.

This section presents (i) a listing of nationally notifiable infectious diseases for 1996, (ii) a tabulation of selected reportable diseases in the United States from 1985 to 1994, (iii) the geographic distributions of and epidemiologic data on selected infectious diseases, and (iv) the geographic distributions of less common notifiable diseases. Data for this section were extracted from MMWR annual summaries, particularly the 1994 summary (MMWR 43, October 6, 1995, issue no. 53, p. 1–80).

Notifiable Diseases

Nationally Notifiable Infectious Diseases—1996

Anthrax
Botulism
Brucellosis
Chlamydia psittaci
   (psittacosis)
Chlamydia trachomitis
   (genital)
Cholera
Coccidioidomycosis
Cryptosporidiosis
Diphtheria
Encephalitis, California
Encephalitis, eastern equine
Encephalitis, St. Louis
Encephalitis, western equine
Escherichia coli O157:H7
Haemophilus ducreyi
   (chancroid)
Haemophilus influenzae
   (invasive)
Hantavirus pulmonary
   syndrome
Hemolytic uremic syndrome
   (postdiarrheal)
Hepatitis A

Hepatitis B
Hepatitis, C/non-A, non-B
Human immunodeficiency
   virus infection (AIDS)
Human immunodeficiency
   virus infection (pediatric)
Legionellosis
Lyme disease
Malaria
Measles (rubeola)
Mumps
Mycobacterum leprae
   (leprosy, Hansen's
   disease)
Mycobacterium tuberculosis
   (tuberculosis)
Neisseria gonorrhoeae
   (genital)
Neisseria meningitidis
   (disseminated)
Pertussis
Plague
Poliomyelitis (paralytic)
Rabies (animal)
Rabies (human)

(*continued*)

Nationally Notifiable Infectious Diseases—1996 (continued)

Rocky Mountain spotted fever
Rubella (congenital)
Rubella (German measles)
Salmonellosis
Shigellosis
Streptococcal disease (group A, invasive)
Streptococcus pneumoniae (drug resistant)
Syphilis (congenital)
Syphilis (all other stages)
Tetanus
Toxic shock syndrome (staphylococcal)
Toxic shock syndrome (streptococcal)
Trichinosis
Typhoid fever
Yellow fever

Table 8.1 Selected reportable diseases in the United States, 1985–1994

Disease	No. of cases in:									
	1994	1993	1992	1991	1990	1989	1988	1987	1986	1985
Amebiasis	2,983	2,970	2,942	2,989	3,328	3,217	2,860	3,123	3,532	4,433
Anthrax	0	0	0	1	0	0	2	1	0	0
Botulism	143	97	91	114	92	89	84	82	109	122
Brucellosis	119	120	105	104	85	95	96	129	106	153
Cholera	39	18	103	26	6	0	8	6	23	4
Diphtheria	2	0	4	5	4	3	2	3	0	3
Legionellosis	1,615	1,280	1,339	1,317	1,370	1,190	1,085	1,038	948	830
Leprosy	136	187	172	154	198	163	184	238	270	361
Leptospirosis	38	51	54	58	77	93	54	43	41	57
Malaria	1,229	1,411	1,087	1,278	1,292	1,277	1,099	944	1,123	1,049
Pertussis	4,617	6,586	4,083	2,719	4,570	4,157	3,450	2,823	4,195	3,589
Plague	17	10	13	11	2	4	15	12	10	17
Psittacosis	38	60	92	94	113	116	114	98	224	119
Rabies (human)	6	3	1	3	1	1	0	0	0	1
Rocky Mountain spotted fever	465	456	502	628	651	623	609	604	760	714
Tetanus	51	48	45	57	64	53	53	48	64	83
Trichinosis	32	16	41	62	129	30	45	40	39	61
Tularemia	96	132	159	193	152	152	201	214	170	177
Typhoid fever	441	440	414	501	552	460	436	400	362	402

Notifiable Diseases

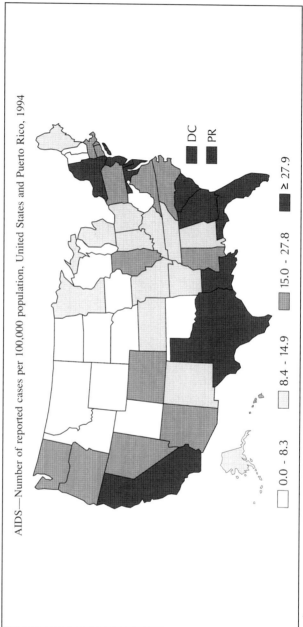

AIDS—Number of reported cases per 100,000 population, United States and Puerto Rico, 1994

DC

PR

0.0 - 8.3   8.4 - 14.9   15.0 - 27.8   ≥ 27.9

Notifiable Diseases

Incidence per 100,000 population

1994–30.1	1993–40.2
1992–17.8	1991–17.3
1990–16.7	1989–13.6
1988–12.6	1987– 8.7
1986– 5.4	1985– 3.5

Percent change since 1985: 860% increase

Demographic factors

Age:

<1 year, 0.4%	1–4 years, 0.5%
5–9 years, 0.2%	10–14 years, 0.2%
15–19 years, 0.4%	20–24 years, 3.3%
25–29 years, 13.0%	30–39 years, 45.3%
40–49 years, 26.4%	50–59 years, 7.6%
60 + years, 2.7%	

Race: Native American, 0.4%; Asian-Pacific, 0.9%; Black, 48.1%; Caucasian, 50.7%

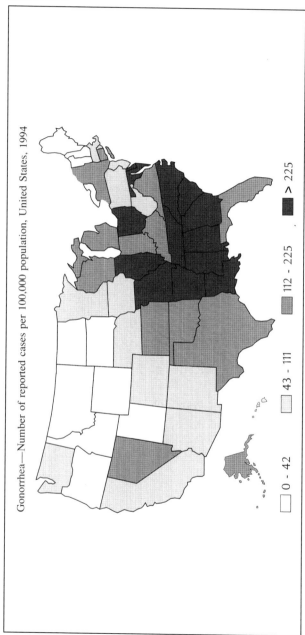

Gonorrhea—Number of reported cases per 100,000 population, United States, 1994

0 - 42   43 - 111   112 - 225   > 225

Notifiable Diseases

Incidence per 100,000 population

1994–168.4	1993–172.4
1992–201.6	1991–249.5
1990–276.6	1989–297.4
1988–298.7	1987–323.1
1986–376.4	1985–384.5

Percent change since 1985: 56.2% decrease

Demographic factors

Age:

10–14 years, 2.1%	15–19 years, 30.6%
20–24 years, 30.1%	25–29 years, 15.0%
30–39 years, 15.9%	40+ years, 6.2%

Race: Native American, 0.6%; Asian-Pacific, 0.5%; Black, 85.3%; Caucasian, 13.7%

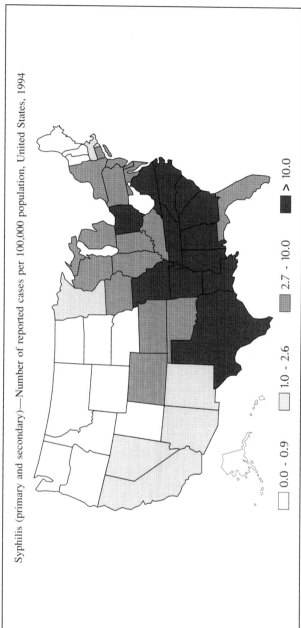

Syphilis (primary and secondary)—Number of reported cases per 100,000 population, United States, 1994

0.0 - 0.9   1.0 - 2.6   2.7 - 10.0   > 10.0

Notifiable Diseases

Incidence per 100,000 population

1994– 8.1	1993–10.4	
1992–13.7	1991–17.3	
1990–20.1	1989–18.1	
1988–16.4	1987–14.5	
1986–11.7	1985–11.5	

Percent change since 1985: 29.6% decrease

Demographic factors

Age: 10–14 years, 0.6% 15–19 years, 10.9%
20–24 years, 19.8% 25–29 years, 18.5
30–39 years, 32.2% 40+ years, 17.9%

Race: Native American, 0.2%; Asian-Pacific, 0.4%; Black, 90.1%; Caucasian, 9.4%

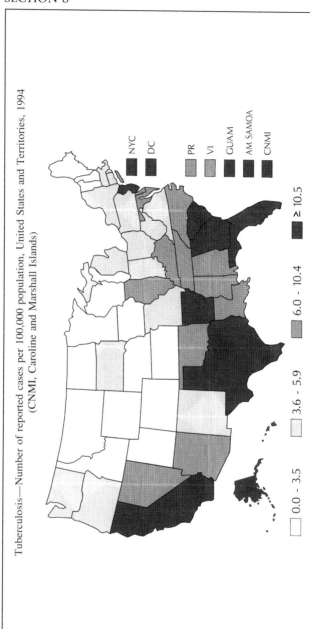

Tuberculosis—Number of reported cases per 100,000 population, United States and Territories, 1994 (CNMI, Caroline and Marshall Islands)

NYC
DC
PR
VI
GUAM
AM SAMOA
CNMI

☐ 0.0 - 3.5   3.6 - 5.9   6.0 - 10.4   ≥ 10.5

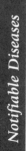

Incidence per 100,000 population

1994– 9.4	1993– 9.8
1992–10.5	1991–10.4
1990–10.3	1989– 9.5
1988– 9.1	1987– 9.3
1986– 9.4	1985– 9.3

Percent change since 1985: 1.1% increase

Demographic factors

Age:
<1 year, 0.7%	1–4 years, 3.5%
5–9 years, 1.6%	10–14 years, 1.1%
15–19 years, 2.2%	20–24 years, 5.3%
25–29 years, 7.4%	30–39 years, 20.0%
40–49 years, 18.0%	50–59 years, 12.0%
60 + years, 28.1%	

Race: Native American, 1.4%; Asian-Pacific, 16.0%; Black, 35.7%; Caucasian, 46.9%

Notifiable Diseases

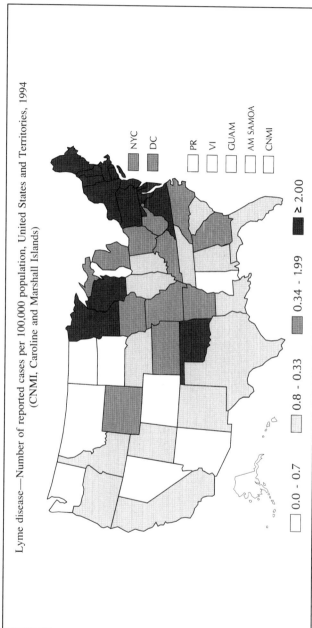

Lyme disease—Number of reported cases per 100,000 population, United States and Territories, 1994 (CNMI, Caroline and Marshall Islands)

NYC
DC

PR
VI
GUAM
AM SAMOA
CNMI

0.0 - 0.7   0.8 - 0.33   0.34 - 1.99   ≥ 2.00

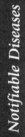

Notifiable Diseases

Incidence per 100,000 population

1994–5.0	1993–3.3
1992–0.1	1991–3.8
	Not reportable before 1991

Demographic factors

Age:

<1 year, 0.2%	1–4 years, 5.1%
5–9 years, 8.9%	10–14 years, 6.5%
15–19 years, 4.9%	20–24 years, 3.7%
25–29 years, 5.0%	30–39 years, 16.1%
40–49 years, 17.2%	50–59 years, 12.9%
60 + years, 19.8%	

Race: Native American, 0.4%; Asian-Pacific, 0.8%; Black, 2.1%; Caucasian, 96.7%

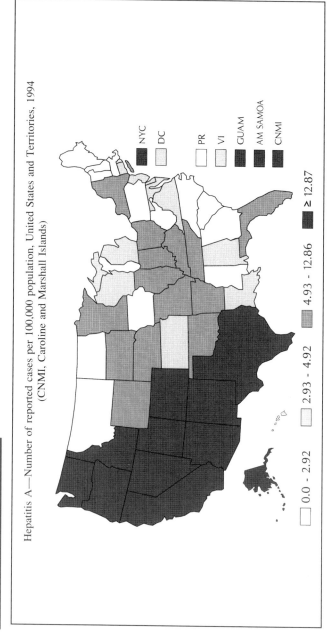

Hepatitis A—Number of reported cases per 100,000 population, United States and Territories, 1994 (CNMI, Caroline and Marshall Islands)

NYC
DC

PR
VI
GUAM
AM SAMOA
CNMI

0.0 - 2.92   2.93 - 4.92   4.93 - 12.86   ≥ 12.87

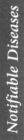

Notifiable Diseases

Incidence per 100,000 population

1994–10.3	1993– 9.4
1992– 9.1	1991– 9.7
1990–12.6	1989–14.4
1988–11.6	1987–10.4
1986–10.0	1985–10.0

Percent change since 1985: 3% increase

Demographic factors

Age: <1 year, 0.5%   1–4 years, 7.3%
        5–9 years, 15.7%   10–14 years, 9.6%
        15–19 years, 7.8%   20–24 years, 10.7%
        25–29 years, 11.5%   30–39 years, 18.9%
        40–49 years, 9.2%   50–59 years, 4.0%
        60+ years, 4.9%

Race: Native American, 11.8%; Asian-Pacific, 2.0%; Black, 8.8%; Caucasian, 77.4%

Notifiable Diseases

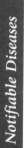

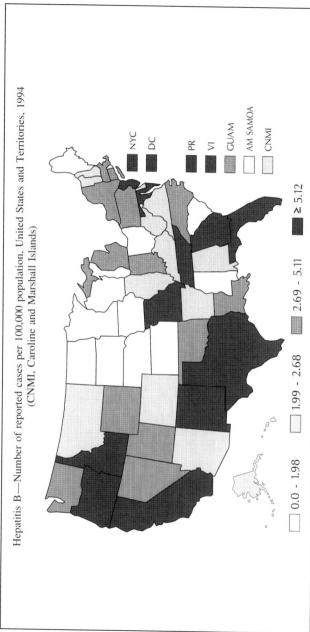

Hepatitis B—Number of reported cases per 100,000 population, United States and Territories, 1994 (CNMI, Caroline and Marshall Islands)

NYC
DC
PR
VI
GUAM
AM SAMOA
CNMI

0.0 - 1.98   1.99 - 2.68   2.69 - 5.11   ≥ 5.12

Incidence per 100,000 population

1994– 4.8	1993– 5.2
1992– 6.3	1991– 7.1
1990– 8.5	1989– 9.4
1988– 9.4	1987–10.7
1986–11.2	1985–11.5

Percent change since 1985: 58.3% decrease

Demographic factors

Age:	<1 year, 0.5%	1–4 years, 0.6%
	5–9 years, 0.7%	10–14 years, 1.4%
	15–19 years, 6.7%	20–24 years, 13.4%
	25–30 years, 16.1%	31–39 years, 30.0%
	40–49 years, 16.8%	50–59 years, 7.0%
	60+ years, 7.0%	

Race: Native American, 1.1%; Asian-Pacific, 9.5%; Black, 31.1%; Caucasian, 58.3%

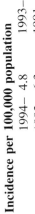

Notifiable Diseases

Geographic Distribution of Less Common Notifiable Diseases—Totals for 1990–1994

Amebiasis
California, 6,361; New York City, 2,470; Texas, 529; Oregon, 528; New York State, 496; Georgia, 407

Botulism
California, 196; Texas, 41; Alaska, 29; Pennsylvania, 29; Washington State, 23

Brucellosis
Texas, 144; California, 143; North Carolina, 56; Illinois, 27; Florida, 22; Georgia, 14

Cholera
California, 90; New Jersey, 13; Texas, 12; New York City, 11

Diphtheria
California, 5; New Mexico, 3; Florida, 2; Kentucky, Pennsylvania, and Minnesota, 1 each

Legionellosis
Ohio, 727; Pennsylvania, 695; New York State, 545; California, 382; Maryland, 268; Wisconsin, 268; Florida, 229; Massachusetts, 223; Georgia, 222; New Jersey, 202; New York City, 200

Leprosy
California, 295; Texas, 189; Hawaii, 91; New York City, 75; Washington State, 45; Massachusetts, 32; Florida, 23

Leptospirosis
Hawaii, 159; Puerto Rico, 31; Missouri, 11; Illinois, 11; Louisiana, 10

Malaria
California, 1,389; New York City, 648; New York State, 348; Texas, 341; Maryland, 315; New Jersey, 299; Florida, 277; North Carolina, 229; Illinois, 212; Massachusetts, 192

Pertussis
California, 2,460; Massachusetts, 1,958; Wisconsin, 1,361; New York State, 1,319; Ohio, 1,156; Pennsylvania, 1,043; Illinois, 1,027; Washington State, 848; Colorado, 805

Plague
New Mexico, 21; Arizona, 10; Colorado, 8; Utah, 4; Idaho, 2; Nevada, Texas, Oklahoma, Maryland, and California, 1 each

Notifiable Diseases

Rabies (Human)
Texas, 4; California, 3; New York State, West Virginia, Georgia, Florida, Tennessee, Alabama, and Arkansas, 1 each

Rocky Mountain Spotted Fever
North Carolina, 624; Oklahoma, 322; Tennessee, 233; Georgia, 200; Missouri, 127; South Carolina, 119; Arkansas, 118; West Virginia, 108; Maryland, 94; Ohio, 88

Tetanus
Texas, 41; California, 29; Florida, 20; Michigan, 17; Puerto Rico, 12; Minnesota, 10; Maryland, 9; Pennsylvania, Indiana, Illinois, and Tennessee, 8 each

Trichinosis
Iowa, 80; Wisconsin, 41; Alaska, 40; California, 18; Virginia, 17; New York State, 15

Tularemia
Arkansas, 181; Missouri, 152; Oklahoma, 51; South Dakota, 39; Montana, 29; Tennessee, 27; Kansas, 24; Colorado, 23

Typhoid Fever
California, 626; New York City, 386; Florida, 151; Illinois, 148; Massachusetts, 119; New Jersey, 113; Texas, 107; New York State, 102

Bibliography

For more detailed information regarding the subjects covered in this pocket guide, please refer to the following general reference texts.

Atlas, R., and L. Parks. 1993. *Handbook of Microbiological Media.* CRC Press, Inc., Boca Raton, Fla.

Balows, A., H. Trüper, M. Dworkin, W. Harder, and K. H. Schleifer. 1992. *The Prokaryotes,* 2nd ed. Springer-Verlag, New York.

Baron, E., L. Peterson, and S. Finegold. 1994. *Bailey & Scott's Diagnostic Microbiology,* 9th ed. Mosby-Year Book, Inc., St. Louis.

Garcia, L. S., and D. A. Bruckner. 1993. *Diagnostic Medical Parasitology,* 2nd ed. American Society for Microbiology, Washington, D.C.

Holt, J., N. Krieg, P. Sneath, J. Staley, and S. Williams. 1994. *Bergey's Manual of Determinative Bacteriology,* 9th ed. The Williams & Wilkins Co., Baltimore.

Isenberg, H. 1992. *Clinical Microbiology Procedures Handbook.* American Society for Microbiology, Washington, D.C.

Kucers, A., and N. M. Bennett. 1989. *The Use of Antibiotics,* 4th ed. J. B. Lippincott Co., Philadelphia.

Kwon-Chung, K., and J. Bennett. 1992. *Medical Mycology.* Lea & Febiger, Philadelphia.

Larone, D. 1995. *Medically Important Fungi—A Guide to Identification,* 3rd ed. American Society for Microbiology, Washington, D.C.

Lorian, V. 1991. *Antibiotics in Laboratory Medicine,* 3rd ed. The Williams & Wilkins Co., Baltimore.

Mandell, G., J. Bennett, and R. Dolin. 1995. *Principles and Practice of Infectious Diseases,* 4th ed. Churchill Livingstone, New York.

Miller, J. M. 1996. *A Guide to Specimen Management in Clinical Microbiology.* American Society for Microbiology, Washington, D.C.

Murray, P. R., E. J. Baron, M. A. Pfaller, F. C. Tenover, and R. H. Yolken. 1995. *Manual of Clinical Microbiology,* 6th ed. American Society for Microbiology, Washington, D.C.

Murray, P. R., G. Kobayashi, M. Pfaller, and K. Rosenthal. 1994. *Medical Microbiology,* 2nd ed. Mosby-Year Book, Inc., St. Louis.

Rose, N. R., E. Conway DeMacario, J. L. Fahey, H. Friedman, and G. M. Penn. 1992. *Manual of Clinical Laboratory Immunology,* 4th ed. American Society for Microbiology, Washington, D.C.

Summanen, P., E. Baron, D. Citron, C. Strong, H. Wexler, and S. Finegold. 1993. *Wadsworth Anaerobic Bacteriology Manual,* 5th ed. Star Publishing Co., Belmont, Calif.

NOTES

NOTES